INTRAUTERINE GROWTH RETARDATION
A Practical Approach

INTRAUTERINE GROWTH RETARDATION
A Practical Approach

Thomas L. Gross, M.D.
Associate Professor and Chairman
Department of Obstetrics and Gynecology
University of Illinois College of Medicine at Peoria
Director of Maternal-Fetal Medicine
St. Francis Medical Center
Peoria, Illinois

Robert J. Sokol, M.D.
Professor and Chairman
Department of Obstetrics and Gynecology
Wayne State University School of Medicine
Chief, Department of Obstetrics and Gynecology
Hutzel Hospital
Detroit, Michigan

YEAR BOOK MEDICAL PUBLISHERS, INC.
CHICAGO • LONDON • BOCA RATON

1 2 3 4 5 6 7 8 9 0 VR 93 92 91 90 89

Library of Congress Cataloging-in-Publication Data

Intrauterine growth retardation: a practical approach/[edited by]
Thomas L. Gross, Robert J. Sokol.
p. cm.
Includes bibliographies and index.
ISBN 0-8151-4006-1
1. Fetus—Growth retardation. I. Gross, Thomas L. II. Sokol, Robert J.
[DNLM: 1. Fetal Growth Retardation. WQ 211 I6185]
RG629.G76I56 1989 88-27642
618.3'2—dc19 CIP
DNLM/DLC
for Library of Congress

Sponsoring Editor: James D. Ryan
Assistant Director, Manuscript Services: Fran Perveiler
Production Project Manager: Gayle Paprocki
Proofroom Manager: Shirley E. Taylor

To our parents,
Gilbert and Anna
Eli and Mildred

CONTRIBUTORS

José M. Belizán, M.D., Ph.D
Centro Rosarino de Estudios Perinatales
Rosario, Argentina

Richard A. Bronsteen, M.D.
Assistant Professor
Division of Maternal-Fetal Medicine
Wayne State University School of Medicine
Grace Hospital
Detroit, Michigan

Mitchell P. Dombrowski, M.D.
Assistant Professor
Division of Maternal-Fetal Medicine
Wayne State University School of Medicine
Hutzel Hospital
Detroit, Michigan

Mark I. Evans, M.D.
Director, Division of Reproductive Genetics
Wayne State University School of Medicine
Hutzel Hospital
Detroit, Michigan

Avroy A. Fanaroff, M.B., F.R.C.P.E.
Professor and Vice Chairman
Department of Pediatrics
Case Western Reserve University School of Medicine
Director of Neonatal Nurseries
Rainbow Babies and Childrens Hospital of University Hospitals of Cleveland
Cleveland, Ohio

Steven H. Golde, M.D.
Perinatologist, St. Joseph Medical Center
Burbank, California

Peter A. T. Grannum, M.D.
Associate Professor
Director of Medical Studies
Department of Obstetrics and Gynecology
Yale University School of Medicine
Director of High Risk Obstetrics
Yale-New Haven Hospital
New Haven, Connecticut

Thomas L. Gross, M.D.
Associate Professor and Chairman
Department of Obstetrics and Gynecology
University of Illinois College of Medicine at Peoria
Director of Maternal-Fetal Medicine
St. Francis Medical Center
Peoria, Illinois

Maureen Hack, M.B., Ch.B.
Associate Professor of Pediatrics
Case Western Reserve University School of Medicine
Neonatologist, Rainbow Babies and Childrens Hospital of University Hospitals of Cleveland
Cleveland, Ohio

Nadya J. Kazzi, M.D.
Assistant Professor of Pediatrics
Wayne State University School of Medicine
Associate Neonatologist
Hutzel Hospital
Detroit, Michigan

Robert M. Kliegman, M.D.
Associate Professor of Pediatrics
Case Western Reserve University School of Medicine
Associate Director of Neonatal Intensive Care Unit
Rainbow Babies and Childrens Hospital of University Hospitals of Cleveland
Cleveland, Ohio

Donald L. Levy, M.D.
Professor and Director
Division of Maternal-Fetal Medicine
Eastern Virginia Medical School
Santara Norfolk General Hospital
Norfolk, Virginia

Federico E. Mariona, M.D.
Clinical Professor of Obstetrics and Gynecology
Wayne State University School of Medicine
Oakwood Hospital
Dearborn, Michigan

Ronald L. Poland, M.D.
Professor of Pediatrics
Wayne State University School of Medicine
Director of Neonatal Services
Detroit Medical Center Affiliated Hospitals
Detroit, Michigan

Robert Resnik, M.D.
Professor and Chairman
Department of Reproductive Medicine
University of California at San Diego School of Medicine
San Diego, California

Vincent L. Smeriglio, Ph.D.
Associate Professor
Department of Maternal and Child Health
The Johns Hopkins University School of Hygiene and Public Health
Baltimore, Maryland

Robert J. Sokol, M.D.
Professor and Chairman
Department of Obstetrics and Gynecology
Wayne State University School of Medicine
Chief, Department of Obstetrics and Gynecology
Hutzel Hospital
Detroit, Michigan

José Villar, M.D., M.P.H., M.Sc.
Associate Professor
Department of Obstetrics and Gynecology
The Johns Hopkins University School of Medicine
Epidemiologist, Prevention Research Program
National Institute of Child Health and Human Development
Baltimore, Maryland

Steven L. Warsof, M.D.
Assistant Professor
Division of Maternal-Fetal Medicine
Eastern Virginia Medical School
Santara Norfolk General Hospital
Norfolk, Virginia

Robert A. Welch, M.D.
Assistant Professor
Department of Obstetrics and Gynecology
Wayne State University School of Medicine
Hutzel Hospital
Detroit, Michigan

Honor M. Wolfe, M.D.
Assistant Professor
Division of Maternal-Fetal Medicine
Wayne State University School of Medicine
Hutzel Hospital
Detroit, Michigan

FOREWORD

Despite our enhanced understanding of fetal physiology and the pathogenesis of many diseases complicating pregnancy, a common problem, intrauterine growth retardation (IUGR), has remained somewhat of an enigma. One of the reasons that the condition is so difficult to characterize is that the definition of IUGR is based on mean weight for gestation. Even if a uniform definition of the fifth percentile (or below) were agreed upon, those fetuses/infants falling below this threshold would include 5% of the normal population. The abnormal infants in this group have a very high perinatal mortality rate and are at increased risk of perinatal asphyxia and neonatal morbidity. Earlier studies also suggest that many growth retarded babies will ultimately be neurologically compromised.

In order to circumvent this inherent mortality and morbidity, the diagnosis must be made early in pregnancy and those fetuses that need increased attention must be identified. Today, it is not difficult to diagnose the undergrown fetus. In fact, with ultrasound it is not only possible to estimate fetal weight with reasonable accuracy, but to determine, by analysis of biometric data, whether the fetus is symmetrically or asymmetrically small. Since the small-for-dates fetuses that contribute most to perinatal mortality are those who are either anomalous, suffering from congenital infection, or are simply deprived, the thrust of today's diagnostic endeavors has been to identify these fetuses.

Improvement in ultrasound technology has allowed us to better diagnose fetal anomalies. Better understanding of congenital infections has enabled investigators to better identify the fetus whose primary growth curtailment is due to infection. Doppler ultrasound investigation has shown promise in singling out the small-for-dates fetus suffering from a faulty supply line. In addition, since many growth-retarded fetuses are hypoxic, it is hoped that percutaneous fetal blood sampling will provide a way to identify and treat the hypoxic fetus, often by timely delivery.

This comprehensive text chronicles the advances made in the last few years in our understanding of the various processes responsible for IUGR and provides an up-to-date version of the diagnosis and treatment of this potentially devastating problem.

John Hobbins, M.D.
Department of Obstetrics and Gynecology
Yale University
New Haven, Connecticut

PREFACE

This textbook is for clinicians only. It is intended to serve as a handbook for students and residents and as an update for the practicing physician on current standard management for intrauterine growth retardation. The scope of the book is broad, and readers with primary obstetric and pediatric interest will find it of value. The manuscript was written and edited to emphasize the clinical aspects and present an outline of the state-of-the-art management for the mother, the growth retarded fetus, and the small-for-gestational-age neonate and infant.

The book is divided into four parts: (1) why fetal growth retardation is important, (2) etiology and mechanisms, (3) diagnostic approaches, and (4) management. Part I defines fetal growth, normal and abnormal. Part II includes chapters reviewing the increased risk to the growth retarded fetus and neonate and, in addition, reviews the conflicting data regarding the long-term risk for abnormal neurodevelopmental outcome in the infant. Part III deals with etiology and includes chapters regarding maternal and placental causes and those associated with intrinsic fetal disease. In Part IV the diagnosis of fetal growth retardation is initially introduced from the standpoint of the clinical history and physical. The major diagnostic tool, i.e., prenatal ultrasound, is covered in detail in Chapter 10. Chapter 10 and its accompanying appendices include all of the information and growth tables needed for the physician to perform Level I ultrasound. A chapter on Doppler blood flow (Chapter 11) is included because of the rapidly expanding knowledge regarding fetal and umbilical blood flow and its relationship to growth retardation. Part V covers the approach to the management of intrauterine growth retardation: the maternal and fetal aspects in Chapters 12 and 13 and the neonatal in Chapter 14.

Chapter 14 gives the clinician caring for high risk newborns a standard approach to reduce morbidity in the small-for-gestational-age neonate from the delivery room to the intensive care nursery. Finally, as the book was being prepared two chapters were added to keep readers current on new concepts. Chapter 15 examines new ideas in invasive fetal therapy, and Chapter 17 reviews the ever present malpractice risk as it relates to the management of intrauterine growth retardation.

The rapid increase in our knowledge regarding antepartum, intrapartum, and neonatal risk in the growth retarded fetus and neonate has raised clinical suspicion to a high level so that ultrasound diagnosis can now allow us to recognize most cases of fetal growth retardation prior to delivery. Of course, once the diagnosis of growth retardation is suspected, we need to search for an etiology. Even if it is not found, we now know that the general application of an intensive care approach both prior to labor and around the time of delivery can allow us to optimize outcome. This book has been edited to help the practicing clinician understand how to perform this intensive care management so that the fetal and neonatal outcome can be raised to the highest possible level.

Thomas L. Gross, M.D.

ACKNOWLEDGMENT

We wish to express our deep appreciation to Irene Nafziger for organizing, editing, typing, and proofreading the entire manuscript.

Thomas L. Gross, M.D.

CONTENTS

PART IV DIAGNOSTIC APPROACHES

PART V MANAGEMENT

PART VI MEDICOLEGAL

PART I

Introduction

1

Definition of Fetal Growth: Normal and Abnormal

Steven H. Golde, M.D.

> Growth is the only evidence of life. . . John Henry Cardinal Newman, Apologia pro Vita Sua, 1864.

Growth is a basic fundamental of life. DNA replicates, cells enlarge and divide, tissues increase in mass, and organisms increase in size and weight. This constant drive to grow is no more evident than in the developing mammalian fetus. Structures form during embryogenesis in a strict sequence encoded by genes and guided by the physical and biochemical environment that surrounds them. Cellular change occurs and is balanced by the generation of new cells, each process keenly dependent on complex interactions between nature and nurture. The identification of growth disturbance would seem a field fully matured, with definitions that are concise and rigorously laid out. Such is not the case. As late as 1966 a major textbook in obstetrics declared that "healthy full-term children frequently weigh less than 3200 g and sometimes as little as 2300 g (5 pounds), although when the weight falls below 2500 g the child is premature *by definition.*"[1] The definition of gestational age in terms of neonatal weight stemmed from the recommendation of the American Academy of Pediatrics in 1935 and was designed to allow data comparisons between urban and impoverished rural areas. Growth, the underlying truth of biology, has been poorly studied in the human.

Since the abandonment of the concept that weight determines age, a host of terms have evolved to describe infants who demonstrate altered growth. Such terms as "small for gestational age" (SGA), "large for gestational age"

(LGA), and "intrauterine growth retardation" (IUGR) have served to focus attention on the special problems of infants with growth disturbance. Such shorthand terms, while focusing attention on a group at risk, may hide significant facts from analysis. Terminology is a double-edged sword serving first to categorize, then to explain a phenomenon. It is the purpose of this chapter to explore the definition of growth and its disturbance, point out current limitations in categorization, and offer some guidelines to categorization that may serve a broader diagnostic and therapeutic purpose.

CELLULAR GROWTH

Tissue growth is characterized by the processes of cell hyperplasia and hypertrophy. Both processes may occur in isolation or in concert. DNA content reaches a maximum before organ weight, suggesting that cell division stops within organs before growth stops.[2] Hyperplasia is a function of the rate of cell division. The higher the rate the greater the amount of tissue generated; hence the larger the animal. Studies conducted in rabbits showed that embryos of larger strains had greater cell numbers at any given point in development than did embryos of smaller strains, and also demonstrated higher rates of mitosis.[3,4]

Hyperplasia and hypertrophy are orchestrated by genetic and environmental influences throughout development and act in three distinct phases. During early fetal growth organ DNA content increases at the same rate as organ protein content. Growth thus is achieved by hyperplasia alone, because the ratio of DNA (a measure of cell number) to protein (a measure of cell size) remains constant. DNA synthesis then slows, but protein production continues at its previous rate. During this period hyperplasia and hypertrophy occur together. Finally, DNA synthesis stops, but net protein synthesis continues, an index of growth by hypertrophy alone.[5]

Insults occurring during these different growth phases are likely to have differing results. Malnourishment, hypoxia, chemical interaction, or all three, if present during the phase of hypertrophic growth, yield smaller offspring in rats, which then are capable of catch-up growth because their cell number remains undisturbed, but cell size is reduced. The cells "fatten" when nutrition is restored.[6,7] These same factors, if present during a period of hyperplastic growth, result in a decreased cell population that is unable to catch up if nutrients are supplied later.[8,9]

RATE OF HUMAN FETAL GROWTH

The rate of organism growth is determined by the sequence of organ system development and varies throughout gestation. Total growth is slow while organs are forming during the first 2 months of fetal life. Growth accelerates sharply by the eighth week, and reaches maximum between 4 and 6 months. Slowing of growth occurs after this time, and remains fairly constant until 3 months of postnatal life.[10]

The mechanisms directing growth are not well understood. Genetics plays a large role. By 1889 Sir Frances Galton recognized that there was a constancy in the stature of populations, independent of differences in upbringing and correlating with mid-parental height.[11] It is currently believed that genetic regulation of stature is polygenic, with at least some of the genes located on both the X and Y chromosomes. Females are smaller than males, weighing on average 150 gm less at term than their male counterparts,[12] and their growth is ultimately more constrained.[13,14]

Though important in determining ultimate size, genetic growth potential is not especially critical in influencing size at birth. Infant birth weight correlates well with maternal weight but only poorly with weight of the father.[15] This was made obvious by the studies of Walton and Hammond[16] on cross-breeding of Shetland ponies and shire horses. Shire mares bred to Shetland stallions gave birth to foals three times larger than foals delivered from Shetland mares bred to shire stallions.

Women who are nutritionally deprived and thus small deliver infants who are also small.[17] There is also good correlation between maternal weight gain and birth weight.[18] The size of the placenta itself may serve to restrict fetal growth. If the fetal-placental weight ratio is compared, the growth-retarded fetus tends to be heavier in relation to the weight of the placenta,[19–21] suggesting that placental growth is impaired first. In contrast to growth-retarded fetuses, twin fetuses are lighter in relation to their placentas than would be expected.[22,23] Growth restriction in these cases may more relate to spatial constraints than to nutrient restriction.[24] Such spatial restriction may also account for the smaller size of firstborn infants.[25]

DEFINITIONS OF HUMAN FETAL GROWTH RETARDATION

Numerous attempts have been made to define populations at risk for adverse outcome due to measured growth disturbances. An early attempt by Battaglia and Lubchenco[26] demonstrated that birth weight and gestational age assessment at birth could be combined to demarcate infants at increased risk. This technique has been used to describe abnormal intrauterine growth and is carried out as follows. The neonate undergoes a physical and neurologic examination in which the factors examined are given points. The scoring has been empirically correlated with a gestational age. The gestational age obtained is then plotted on a nomogram along with the birth weight. Various levels have been used to define fetal growth retardation, including less than the 2.5th, 5th, or 10th birth weight percentile. The definitions most frequently

ESTIMATION OF GESTATIONAL AGE BY MATURITY RATING

Symbols: X - 1st Exam O - 2nd Exam

NEUROMUSCULAR MATURITY

	0	1	2	3	4	5
Posture						
Square Window (Wrist)	90°	60°	45°	30°	0°	
Arm Recoil	180°		100°-180°	90°-100°	< 90°	
Popliteal Angle	180°	160°	130°	110°	90°	< 90°
Scarf Sign						
Heel to Ear						

Gestation by Dates __________ wks

Birth Date __________ Hour __________ am pm

APGAR __________ 1 min __________ 5 min

MATURITY RATING

Score	Wks
5	26
10	28
15	30
20	32
25	34
30	36
35	38
40	40
45	42
50	44

PHYSICAL MATURITY

	0	1	2	3	4	5
SKIN	gelatinous red, trans-parent	smooth pink, visible veins	superficial peeling &/or rash, few veins	cracking pale area, rare veins	parchment, deep cracking, no vessels	leathery, cracked, wrinkled
LANUGO	none	abundant	thinning	bald areas	mostly bald	
PLANTAR CREASES	no crease	faint red marks	anterior transverse crease only	creases ant. 2/3	creases cover entire sole	
BREAST	barely percept.	flat areola, no bud	stippled areola, 1–2 mm bud	raised areola, 3–4 mm bud	full areola, 5–10 mm bud	
EAR	pinna flat, stays folded	sl. curved pinna, soft with slow recoil	well-curv. pinna, soft but ready recoil	formed & firm with instant recoil	thick cartilage, ear stiff	
GENITALS Male	scrotum empty, no rugae		testes descend-ing, few rugae	testes down, good rugae	testes pendulous, deep rugae	
GENITALS Female	prominent clitoris & labia minora		majora & minora equally prominent	majora large, minora small	clitoris & minora completely covered	

SCORING SECTION

	1st Exam=X	2nd Exam=O
Estimating Gest Age by Maturity Rating	______ Weeks	______ Weeks
Time of Exam	Date ______ Hour ______ am pm	Date ______ Hour ______ am pm
Age at Exam	______ Hours	______ Hours
Signature of Examiner	______ M.D.	______ M.D.

FIG 1–1.
Modified Dubowitz examination scoring sheet for determining pediatric estimate of gestational age. (Courtesy of Bristol Myers USPNG, Evansville, Indiana.)

used clinically are SGA—less than or equal to the 10th birth weight percentile—and LGA—equal to or higher than the 90th birth weight percentile (Fig 1–1). Although this is a very useful scheme and the most frequently used clinical method for defining fetal growth retardation, there are major sources of potential error. The data used to define the original growth curves were generated in a population at high altitude, an environment that may produce slower fetal growth. Other investigators have since redefined SGA neonates in their own populations near sea level, and these studies find that the data from the high altitudes often exclude 30% to 50% of neonates defined as SGA at sea level. Another major problem is that constitutionally small infants such as those normally born to small parents are classified as SGA by this method. In spite of these drawbacks, Battaglia and Lubchenco's method of defining fetal growth retardation remains the most commonly used in clinical practice.[26]

SYMMETRIC AND ASYMMETRIC GROWTH RETARDATION

Gruenwald[22] compared fetal birth weights in terms of standard deviation from the mean. In 1963 Gruenwald distinguished between acute distress seen among fetuses during labor and a state of "chronic fetal distress" that exists in growth-retarded fetuses for a variable period before onset of labor.[27] He identified two distinct patterns of slowed growth—asymmetric and symmetric—based on how long the growth-altering factor had been present.[27] In the asymmetric type, growth of the fetal trunk is retarded compared with that of the head (relative brain sparing); in the symmetric pattern, growth of the entire fetus is restricted. These patterns roughly correspond to alterations in growth patterns seen in relation to the phase of growth present at the time of the insult.

Symmetric Growth Retardation

Because early phase growth is predominantly by cell hyperplasia, early phase insults tend to irreducibly lower cell number. The entire organism's potential for organ growth is reduced. Trunk and head size are concomitantly limited, and a symmetric pattern of restricted growth is observed. Karyotypic anomalies and transplacental infections are most likely to yield such a pattern.

Asymmetric Growth Retardation

Cell hypertrophy is also affected by these processes, but to a lesser degree than hyperplasia is. Late influences, such as those seen with maternal vascular disease, restrict fetal growth during the predominant hypertrophic growth phase. During this period relative depletion of actively growing liver and subcutaneous fat is affected more than is growth of the fetal brain, resulting in decreased trunk growth compared with linear or head growth. If either process begins early enough or is severe, the patterns may merge and be indistinguishable.

PONDERAL INDEX

Miller and Hassanein[28] described the use of Rohrer's Ponderal Index

$$\frac{\text{Birth weight}}{(\text{Crown-heel length})^3} \times 100$$

in a population of more than 700 neonates to accurately account for differences in symmetry. This method adequately links size to weight in a fashion that identifies patterns of growth failure. In addition, it can differentiate the asymmetrically growth-retarded fetus from those that are normally small due to small parental size. However, it is subject to error because of methodologic problems in obtaining precise neonatal length. Small errors in the measurement of fetal length may make large differences in the calculation of ponderal indices, because the length is cubed. Miller and Merritt[29] later reported that only 5% of full-term white infants (either first or later born) had ponderal indices less than 2.26. Such infants tended to demonstrate catch-up growth postnatally, as expected from an injury leading to arrest of growth during the hypertrophic cell growth phase.[29]

It is clear that fetal growth is complex. The issue is central to any discussion of fetal compromise. Patterns of normal growth are poorly defined in the literature and normative data are lacking. Few studies sufficiently restrict data to normal populations. End points measured to date have been imprecise and limited. Techniques to gauge growth in the fetus are expanding, with a wider appreciation of the importance of patterns of fetal growth and improvements in equipment. Graphic analysis of multiple morphometric measures offers greater precision in gestational dating[30] and a realization of individualized growth rate assessment. With greater use of rate-descriptive fetal ultrasonography and more attention to proper classification of neonatal growth in the nursery, improvement in the definition of retarded growth is inevitable.

REFERENCES

1. Eastman NJ, Hellman LM, Pritchard JA: *Williams Obstetrics,* ed 13. New York, Appleton-Century-Crofts, 1966.
2. Enesco M, Le Blond CP: Increase in cell number as a factor in the growth of the organs of the young male rat. *J Embryol Exp Morphol* 1962; 10:530.
3. Castle WE, Gregory PW: The embryological basis of size inheritance in the rabbit. *J Morphol Physiol* 1929; 48:81.
4. Gregory PW, Castle WE: Further studies on the embryological basis of size inheritance in the rabbit. *J Exp Zool* 1931; 59:199.
5. Winick M, Noble A: Quantitative changes in ribonucleic acids and protein during normal growth of rat placenta. *Nature* 1966; 212:34.
6. Widdowson EM, McCance RA: A review: New thoughts on growth. *Pediatr Res* 1975; 9:154.
7. Prader A, Tanner JM, Harnack GA: Catch-up following illness or starvation. *J Pediatr* 1963; 62:646.
8. Winick M, Noble A: Cellular response in rats during malnutrition at various ages. *J Nutr* 1966; 89:300.
9. Fish I, Winick M: Cellular growth in various regions of the developing rat brain. *Pediatr Res* 1969; 3:407.

10. Thompson DW: *On Growth and Form.* Cambridge, Cambridge University Press, 1942.
11. Galton F: *Natural Inheritance.* New York, Macmillan Publishing Co, 1889.
12. Klossterman GJ: On intrauterine growth: The significance of prenatal care. *Int J Gynaecol Obstet* 1970; 8:895.
13. Garn SM, Rohmann CG: Variability in the order of ossification of the body centers of the hand and wrist. *Am J Phys Anthropol* 1960; 18:219.
14. Garn SM, Rohmann CG: X-linked inheritance of developmental timing in man. *Nature* 1962; 196:695.
15. Cawley RH, McKeown T, Record RG: Parental stature and birth weight. *Am J Hum Genet* 1954; 6:448.
16. Walton A, Hammond J: The maternal effects on growth and conformation in the Shire horse-Shetland pony crosses. *Proc R Soc Lond [Biol]* 1938; 125:311.
17. Lechtig A, Yarbough C, Delgado H, et al: Effect of moderate maternal malnutrition on the placenta. *Am J Obstet Gynecol* 1975; 123:191.
18. Simpson JW, Lawless RW, Mitchell AC: The responsibility of the obstetrician to the fetus. *Obstet Gynecol* 1975; 45:481.
19. Garow J: The relationship of fetal growth to size and composition of the placenta. *Proc R Soc Med* 1970; 63:498.
20. Thompson AM, Billewicz WZ, Hytten FE: The assessment of fetal growth. *Br J Obstet Gynaecol* 1968; 75:903.
21. Thompson AM, Billewicz WZ, Hytten FE: The weight of the placenta in relation to birth weight. *Br J Obstet Gynaecol* 1969; 76:865.
22. Gruenwald P: Growth of the human fetus. *Am J Obstet Gynecol* 1962; 94:112.
23. McKeown T, Record RG: The influence of placental size on foetal growth in man with special reference to multiple pregnancy. *J Endocrinol* 1953; 9:418.
24. McKeown T, Record RG: Observations on foetal growth in multiple pregnancy in man. *J Endocrinol* 1952; 8:386.
25. Krogman WM: *Child Growth.* Ann Arbor, University of Michigan Press, 1972.
26. Battaglia FC, Lubchenco LO: A practical classification of newborn infants by weight and gestational age. *J Pediatr* 1967; 71:159.
27. Gruenwald P: Chronic fetal distress and placental insufficiency. *Biol Neonate* 1963; 5:215.
28. Miller HC, Hassanein K: Diagnosis of impaired fetal growth in newborn infants. *Pediatrics* 1971; 48:511.
29. Miller HC, Merritt TA: *Fetal Growth in Humans.* Chicago, Year Book Medical Publishers, 1979.
30. Hadlock FP, Deter RL, Harrist RB, et al: Computer assisted analysis of fetal age in the third trimester using multiple fetal growth parameters. *JCU* 1983; 11:313.

PART II

Why Fetal Growth Retardation Is Important

2

Increased Risk to the Growth-Retarded Fetus

Honor M. Wolfe, M.D.
Thomas L. Gross, M.D.

Low birth weight is the primary cause of perinatal mortality and long- and short-term infant morbidity. Improvement in antenatal and neonatal care has resulted in a substantial decrease in perinatal mortality over the past decade. The subset of low birth weight infants, however, is not homogeneous. It is estimated that one third of infants with birth weight less than 2500 gm are not premature but are term infants whose birth weight reflects impaired intrauterine growth. When birth weight is examined with reference to gestational age, prematurity and growth retardation in infants of comparable birth weight are found to be clinically distinct in terms of etiology, prognosis, and risks.

With the declining frequency of disease such as erythroblastosis fetalis and improving survival of premature infants, intrauterine growth retardation is becoming an increasingly significant factor in perinatal mortality. Indeed, growth retardation ranks second to prematurity as a cause of perinatal loss. This chapter addresses the antepartum and intrapartum risks to the infant who is small for gestational age (SGA).

STILLBIRTH

Examination of the fetal mortality rate for SGA infants reveals that the risk of death in utero is significant. Although congenital anomalies are associated with approximately one third of stillbirths among growth-retarded fetuses, asphyxia remains the primary cause of perinatal mortality and morbidity in the SGA infant. In this respect fetal death represents the far extreme of a wide spectrum of uteroplacental insufficiency. It is assumed that, in the absence of congenital anomalies, the stillborn SGA fetus has exhausted its compensatory mechanisms in the face of a nutrient and oxygen supply inadequate to maintain intrauterine life.

Gestational Age

A definite association between impaired intrauterine growth and stillbirth has been noted, but the actual frequency of the association has been obscured by inaccurate recording. The absence of dating parameters, including the Dubowitz assessment, variable and often unknown duration between fetal death and delivery, and the poorly defined effect of maceration on fetal weight make determination of birth weight percentile and growth retardation in stillborn fetuses difficult. Despite these shortcomings, several authors have confirmed the high frequency of stillbirth among SGA fetuses. A study in 1980 by Manara[1] demonstrated that at least 20% of all stillborn fetuses show some degree of growth retardation. Morrison and Olsen,[2] in a study of 765 stillbirths, found hypoxia to be the major cause of intrauterine fetal death, accounting for 43% of stillbirths in their series. Intrauterine growth retardation (IUGR) accounted for 26% of hypoxia-related stillbirths among infants weighing less than 2500 gm. A protocol for diagnosing the cause of intrauterine fetal death and managing the delivery has recently been described.[3]

The gestational age at which fetal death occurs in the growth-retarded fetus is likely a function of both the severity and the duration of the uteroplacental insufficiency. A cross-sectional retrospective review of greater than two million births in California[4] found fetal mortality to rise with advancing gestation in the SGA fetus. Tejani et al.[5] observed that although intrauterine death may occur at any gestational age in the growth-retarded fetus, it is seen mainly in the last 3 to 4 weeks of pregnancy. Five of six, or 83%, of the fetal deaths in their study occurred at or beyond 36 weeks gestation. This confirmed an earlier study by Usher,[6] who found that fetal death, even among severely growth-retarded infants (less than the 3rd birth weight percentile), occurred at or beyond 35 weeks in 21 of 27, or 78%, of the cases in their series.

For nearly all age-weight combinations, neonatal and fetal mortality each comprise 50% of the total perinatal mortality. As can be seen in Figure 2–1, adapted from Williams et al.,[4] perinatal mortality drops with advancing gestational age. The graph demonstrates that at any gestational age pregnancies in which the neonate weighs less than the 10th birth weight percentile were associated with a significantly greater perinatal mortality when compared with pregnancies of comparable gestational age in which the birth weight of the neonate was at the 50th birth weight percentile. Figure 2–2 shows that for any fixed weight perinatal mortality initially decreases with advancing

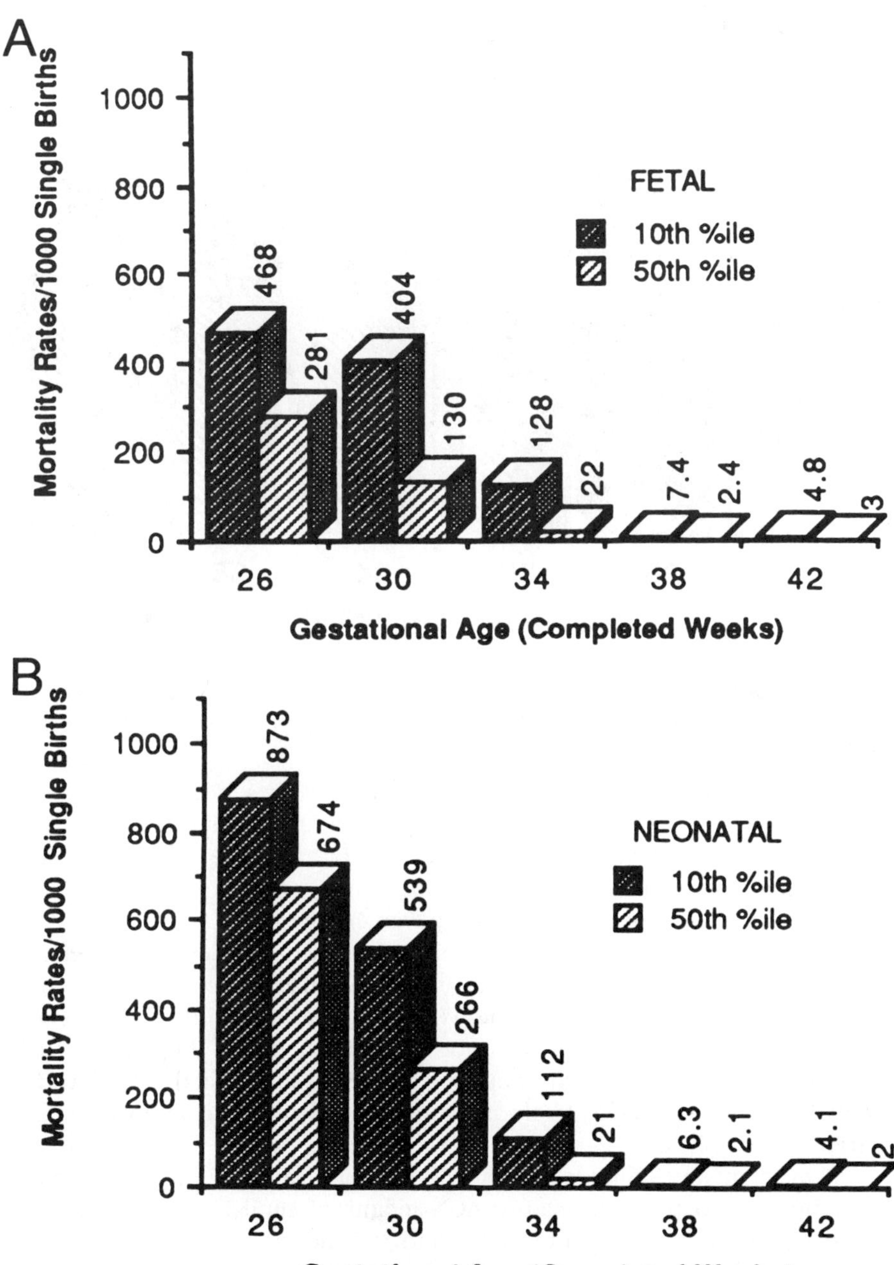

FIG 2–1.
A and **B**, fetal and neonatal mortality rates per 1,000 single births for gestations at the 10th and 50th birth weight percentiles (Adapted from Williams RL, Creasy RK, Cunningham GC, et al: *Obstet Gynecol* 1982; 59:624.)

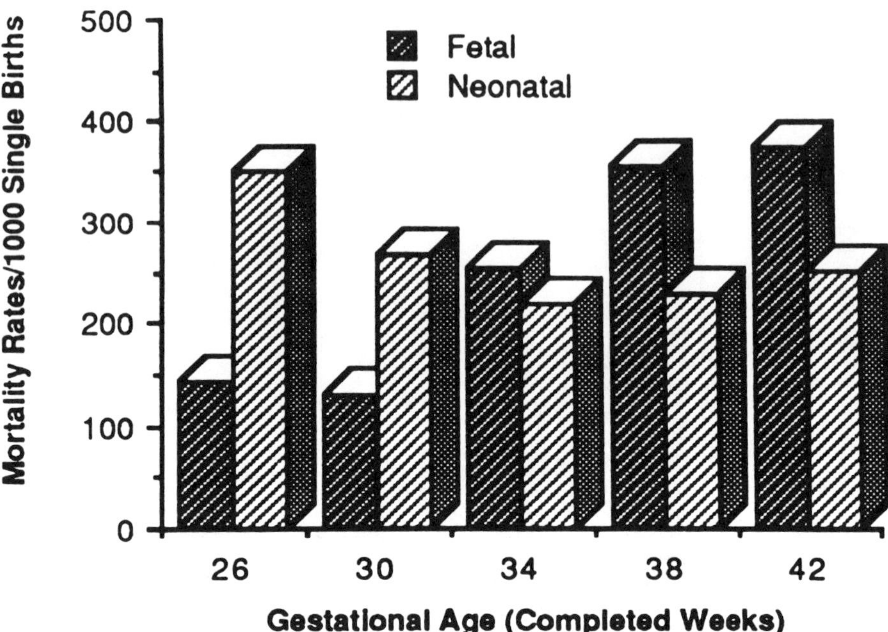

FIG 2–2.
Fetal and neonatal mortality rates for infants weighing 1,350 to 1,500 gm at various gestational ages. (Adapted from Williams RL, Creasy RK, Cunningham GC, et al: *Obstet Gynecol* 1982; 59:624.)

gestation, reaches a minimum, and then again increases. When the two components of perinatal mortality (fetal death and neonatal death) are examined separately, the trend and relative contribution of each differs in the SGA and appropriate for gestational age (AGA) pregnancy.

Fetal mortality rises steadily with advancing gestation in the SGA fetus. The initial drop in perinatal mortality among growth-retarded infants reflects an improving neonatal survival with increasing maturity that until approximately 38 weeks is greater than the worsening rate of fetal deaths. Neonatal mortality among SGA infants does not continue to exhibit the expected fall seen among AGA infants with advancing gestation, and indeed begins to rise between 38 and 42 weeks, likely as a function of worsening antepartum and intrapartum asphyxia.

SGA infants weighing less than 2,500 gm at term have a lower neonatal mortality rate than do premature AGA infants of similar weight. They do, however, exhibit a perinatal mortality 5 to 30 times greater than that of AGA infants at 38 to 42 weeks. It is frequently stated that SGA infants have accelerated maturity and thus improved outcome compared with AGA infants. However, as has been demonstrated, when mortality rates are compared on the basis of gestational age rather than birth weight, the concept of improved outcome among SGA infants shows little validity.

LABOR

In 1963 Gruenwald[7] distinguished between the acute distress seen among fetuses during labor and a state of "chronic fetal distress" that exists in growth-retarded fetuses for a variable period before onset of labor. Normal growth and development in utero depend on the maintenance of fetal homeostasis via metabolic exchanges with the mother through the placenta. Chronic or subacute fetal distress occurs in the growth-retarded fetus when this homeostasis is disturbed under conditions of uteroplacental insufficiency. Decreased nutrient supply from the mother slows the deposition of fat and glycogen stores in the growth-retarded fetus. Impairment of both gas exchange and clearance of fetal metabolites means that the growth-retarded fetus may suffer variable degrees of metabolic acidosis and exhibit chronically low Po_2 prior to the onset of labor. Initial adaptive responses to this deprived intrauterine environment include decreased fetal motion to conserve energy, preferential shunting of the limited blood flow away from fetal viscera and musculature toward the brain and myocardium, and slowed growth in utero. The growth-retarded fetus may enter the third trimester with a decreased reserve, having already exhausted its nutrient supply and many of its adaptive mechanisms, and with chronically low Po_2.

With the onset of uterine contractions, the intramyometrial pressure increases and the uterine muscle fibers act like sphincters, completely surrounding the vessels within the myometrium, leading to their partial or complete occlusion. With the resultant circulatory stasis, blood in the intervillous space has decreased oxygen and fuels, such as glucose, that are continuously used by the fetus. Catabolites, which are continuously produced, accumulate. Therefore during labor, hypoxemia, hypercapnea, and acidosis can be present in the intervillous space and fetal blood. Under conditions of normal fetal reserve the decrease in Po_2 produced by uterine contractions does not reach what Pose et al.[8] refer to as a "critical level," and no decelerations in fetal heart rate are observed even with intense uterine contractions. The growth-retarded fetus, however, enters labor with an abnormally low baseline Po_2 and often some degree of underlying acidosis. The transient reduction of maternal blood flow during contractions can decrease the fetal Po_2 below the critical level and result in decelerated fetal heart rate, hypoxia, and acidosis. Indeed, with progressively worsening hypoxia during labor, the growth-retarded fetus may become dependent on anaerobic metabolism and metabolic acidosis may develop because of the accumulation of lactate.

The importance of impaired fetal reserve is clinically apparent. Even with the shorter and less intense contractions associated with an oxytocin challenge test (OCT), evidence of fetal distress is seen more often in the growth-retarded fetus. In fact, IUGR is the single high-risk condition yielding the greatest number of positive OCT results. Lin et al.[9] found that approximately one third of all positive OCT results were associated with growth-retarded fetuses and that approximately 30% of growth-retarded fetuses (versus 10% of "high risk" non-SGA fetuses) demonstrate positive OCT reactions.

It is not surprising, therefore, that studies of intrapartum fetal heart rate tracings in growth-retarded fetuses demonstrate a significantly greater number of early, variable, and late decelerations.[10] As early as 1965, Dawkins[11] found intrapartum fetal distress to be twice as common in the growth-retarded fetus as in controls. He found that death during labor or immediately after birth was five times more common among SGA infants than in those with normal intrauterine growth. The British Perinatal Study[12] confirmed a fivefold increase in intrapartum fetal death among growth-retarded fetuses compared with their AGA peers.

Variable decelerations are thought to be due primarily to compression of the umbilical cord. There are several hypotheses for the high incidence of variable decelerations in the growth-retarded fetus. Hypoxia often seen in SGA infants reduces the arterial pressure of the cord, making it less turgid and perhaps increasing its susceptibility to compression. The presence of oligohydramnios and possibly an abnormally low concentration of Wharton's jelly may also lead to a cord more easily compressed, with more early decelerations.

Early decelerations are also seen with increased frequency in growth-retarded fetuses. These are thought to be a response to compression of the fetal head. Both the diminished subcutaneous fat and the frequent presence of oligohydramnios may lead to the greater incidence of head compression in the growth-retarded fetus. Of greatest significance, however, is the higher incidence of late decelerations present in the growth-retarded fetus. Late decelerations reflect hypoxia and acidosis and eventually result in myocardial depression.

In addition to demonstrating more ominous fetal heart rate patterns during labor, the growth-retarded fetus exhibits a lower pH for comparable fetal heart rate abnormalities than its AGA counterpart does. Studies have demonstrated that the acidosis reflects an increase in lactate, presumably due to anaerobic metabolism of glucose by the hypoxic fetus.[13] Asphyxia is present more frequently and is more pronounced in infants with IUGR than in infants whose birth weight is greater than the 10th percentile. Lin et al.,[13] in a study of 31 growth-retarded infants, found moderate to severe metabolic acidosis in nearly 50% at delivery. Such fetal compromise occurred more frequently in nulliparous patients, premature deliveries, and pregnancies complicated by severe preeclampsia. However, it is important to note that asphyxia may be associated with growth retardation in the absence of any other maternal medical or obstetric complications.

MECONIUM

Meconium is made up of swallowed amniotic fluid, gastrointestinal secretions, and mucosal cells shed from the lower gastrointestinal tract of the fetus. It is recognized that meconium is passed into the amniotic fluid in about 8% to 15% of all pregnancies either before or during labor. Several high-risk fetal conditions, including growth retardation, prolonged pregnancy, and preeclampsia, have been associated with a significantly greater frequency of meconium passage in utero. Although meconium is associated with increased perinatal morbidity and mortality, its presence does not always indicate a pathologic condition in the fetus and indeed may be physiologic. Causes leading to meconium passage in utero include transient increases in vagal tone resulting, for example, from head or umbilical cord compression. Hypoxia can cause relaxation of the anal sphincter and vasoconstriction in the fetal gut, leading to hyperperistalsis with the passage of meconium. Maturity of the gastrointestinal tract is also known to be important, and meconium is rarely passed in the premature fetus. Numerous studies have addressed the issue of the relative significance of the type of meconium (i.e., thick versus thin) and the time period in which it is passed (i.e., prior to labor versus intrapartum). There is little question, however, that when seen in the growth-retarded fetus, meconium should be considered a sign of asphyxia and fetal distress.

The major risk associated with meconium passage by the growth-retarded fetus is the development of meconium aspiration syndrome (MAS). The overall frequency of symptomatic MAS is 1% to 3%, with a neonatal mortality rate approaching 30%.[14] Even in those infants surviving in MAS, therapy is often prolonged and the hypoxic insult pronounced. Carson et al.[15] therefore recommended that prevention of aspiration is the most effective form of management of MAS.

There are two major periods at which the growth-retarded fetus or infant is at risk for MAS. The first and most common is during delivery. Gregory et al.[16] found a 56% incidence of meconium in the tracheas of infants born with meconium-stained amniotic fluid. Approximately 20% of infants with meconium-stained amniotic fluid or approximately one third of infants with meconium in their tracheas will develop MAS. Inasmuch as fetal gasping in utero is usually not of a frequency or intensity sufficient to transport meconium to the alveoli, the frequency of MAS can be reduced substantially by deep intrapartum suctioning of the nasopharynx after delivery of the infant's head and before delivery of the shoulders. The incidence and severity of MAS are related to both the concentration and the quantity of meconium aspirated. Low concentrations or small amounts of aspirated meconium have not been associated with airway disease in animals. Several factors make the growth-retarded infant at especially high risk for MAS. The frequent occurrence of oligohydramnios in growth-retarded infants will increase the concentration of meconium passed in utero. The higher rate of asphyxia in SGA infants may result in antepartum or intrapartum gasping and a substantial amount of thick meconium present at or below the infant's vocal cords at delivery.[17]

The antepartum period represents a second, small but significant period of risk for MAS.[18] There are many documented cases of asphyxiated fetuses in whom meconium was present in the lungs despite immediate thorough suctioning prior to neonatal respiratory efforts.[19,20] It is postulated that antenatal hypoxia and asphyxia may result in an exaggeration of physiologic respiratory efforts in utero and varying degrees of in utero meconium aspiration.

If meconium aspiration is to be prevented, it is important to recognize that MAS is not solely a neonatal event. Careful intrapartum suctioning will prevent a majority of cases of aspiration at the time of delivery; prevention of fetal asphyxia is necessary to prevent aspiration in utero.

CESAREAN SECTION

Labor adds stress that is poorly tolerated by the growth-retarded fetus. This likely explains the increased risk for operative delivery of growth-retarded infants. When growth retardation is recognized in the antepartum period, cesarean section rates of up to 60% have been reported. Although fetal distress is a frequent indication for cesarean section, a substantial number are elective interventions by the obstetrician. Mann et al.[21] reported that a third of cesarean sections were performed because of cephalopelvic disproportion, which may be related to asymmetric (head sparing) growth retardation or to less severely impaired growth. In addition, the severity of maternal disease sometimes associated with compromised intrauterine growth may prohibit the induction of labor, thereby increasing the rate of cesarean section.

It is of note that the increased risk for cesarean section is primarily among those infants recognized as growth retarded in the antenatal period. In a study of 101 growth-retarded infants, Tejani et al.[5] found an overall cesarean section rate of 21%. Thirty-eight percent of their infants with prenatally diagnosed growth retardation, but only 12% with undiagnosed growth retardation were delivered by cesarean section. The reason for this discrepancy is not clear; it may be a function of heightened physician concern for a fetus recognized to be growth retarded in the antepartum period, or may reflect the fact that those fetuses detected in the antenatal period are the more severely growth retarded and therefore at increased risk for fetal distress and operative intervention during labor.

OLIGOHYDRAMNIOS

Oligohydramnios is relatively uncommon in the general obstetric population, with an overall frequency of approximately 4%.[22] There is no one consistent definition of oligohydramnios, and its frequency therefore will vary based on the criteria used for diagnosis. Oligohydramnios occurs more frequently when the fetus is growth retarded. Decreased amniotic fluid is associated with certain fetal risks, and oligohydramnios accounts for some of the increase in antepartum and intrapartum morbidity and mortality among growth-retarded fetuses.

Association With IUGR

The association of oligohydramnios with fetal growth retardation has recently been recognized. Chamberlain et al.[23] found that the frequency of growth retardation in pregnancies with normal amniotic fluid volume was only 5%; in those with marginally reduced amniotic fluid volume, 20%; and in those with frank oligohydramnios, growth retardation approached 40%. Manning et al.[24] reported that 83% (26 of 31) of the IUGR births in his series were preceded by decreased qualitative amniotic fluid volume. Philipson et al.[22] confirmed a 40% incidence of SGA births in pregnancies complicated with oligohydramnios. He noted that IUGR associated with oligohydramnios tended to occur in pregnancies in young women with hypertension, whereas IUGR in the presence of normal fluid volume was seen in pregnancies in women with a low prepregnancy weight. Although such studies initially suggested the diagnostic value of oligohydramnios for detection of IUGR, its clinical application has been disappointing. When correction is made for the incidence of oligohydramnios and IUGR in the unselected population, Philipson concluded that only 16% of SGA births would be preceded by oligohydramnios. A detailed description of the use of amniotic fluid volume in the detection of IUGR is presented in Chapter 10.

Mechanism

The cause of oligohydramnios in the anatomically normal growth-retarded fetus is likely related to fetal adaptation to hypoxia. With hypoxia there is preferential shunting of oxygen to the brain. In the second half of pregnancy fetal urine and lung fluid are the major contributors to amniotic fluid; thus the drop in renal blood flow and virtual cessation of pulmonary blood flow are believed to result in a marked decline of amniotic fluid production in the pregnancy.

Clinical Risk

Mortality.— Definite clinical risks are associated with oligohydramnios, including increased neonatal and fetal mortality.[25] Even when corrected for congenital anomalies, Chamberlain et al.[23] found a 9.4% incidence of fetal death in pregnancies complicated by oligohydramnios. Overall, corrected perinatal mortality in this study was approximately 50 times higher when oligohydramnios was present.

Congenital Anomalies.—The incidence of major congenital anomalies is significantly related to qualitative amniotic fluid volume. In a study of 7,582 referred high-risk patients, Chamberlain et al.[23] reported the incidence of congenital anomalies to be less than 1% in the presence of normal amniotic fluid volume. Infants with marginally decreased amniotic fluid or frank oligohydramnios showed, respectively, a 2.5% and 9.4% incidence of congenital malformations, including cardiac defects and renal agenesis. Manning et al.[24] found a 13.8% incidence of renal agenesis when oligohydramnios was present in a group of patients with suspected IUGR.

Second-Trimester Oligohydramnios.—Neonatal outcome in the presence of oligohydramnios is related not only to associated congenital anomalies but also to the gestational age at which oligohydramnios develops. Severe oligohydramnios that appears during the second trimester is rare, but when it occurs has been associated with poor fetal prognosis regardless of the cause. Of the 15 case reports of second-trimester oligohydramnios in the literature, only one pregnancy resulted in a living child.[26] There were two spontaneous abortions at 20 weeks, one premature delivery at 22 weeks, seven infants with severe renal anomalies incompatible with extrauterine life, two intrauterine fetal deaths, and two deaths in the immediate neonatal period. A recent literature review has reported that the combination of elevated maternal serum α-fetoprotein and oligohydramnios in the second trimester was associated with a live birth rate of 11%. The surviving neonates were usually growth retarded.[27]

Mechanical and Developmental Effects.—With prolonged, early-onset oligohydramnios the mechanical and developmental effects on the fetus can be profound.[28] There may be temporary positional deformities and contractures. Pulmonary hypoplasia is a potential complication,[29] and is associated with 100% mortality. Meconium, when passed into a decreased volume of amniotic fluid, is thicker and of greater risk to the fetus and neonate from aspiration. Cord compression and cord accidents are also more common with oligohydramnios. Vintzileos et al.[30] in 1983 found decreased amniotic fluid volume in a biophysical profile to be the best predictor of subsequent fetal distress. Manning et al.[24] reported a tenfold increase in fetal distress during labor and neonatal depression in pregnancies complicated by oligohydramnios.

Bottoms et al.[31] concluded that neither subjective sonographic evaluation of amniotic fluid volume nor measurement of maximum vertical pocket alone can accurately predict or rule out the birth of a small, appropriate, or large for gestational age infant in the individual pregnancy. The presence of oligohydramnios, however, should alert the clinician to the possibility of intrauterine hypoxia, congenital malformations, and worsened perinatal outcome, especially when seen in conjunction with suspected IUGR.

GENETICS

Chromosomal anomalies are known to be a cause of abnormal intrauterine and postnatal growth. Genetic effects on growth are discussed in more detail in Chapter 6, and only a summary of the relationship of genetic anomalies and fetal growth retardation is presented here.

The mechanism for growth retardation in chromosomal abnormalities remains speculative. It is estimated that 90% of abnormal conceptuses are lost in spontaneous abortion, leaving an approximately 2% to 3% incidence of major genetic and structural abnormalities present at birth. Because growth failure in utero is a prominent feature of most recognized chromosomal abnormalities and certain structural defects, the relatively small incidence of congenital anomalies is concentrated among SGA infants. Thus major congenital anomalies must be strongly considered in the presence of severe fetal growth retardation.

The conditions most commonly associated with growth retardation include trisomy 13, trisomy 18, and renal agenesis. Growth retardation is also seen with Turner's syndrome, autosomal deletions such as cri du chat syndrome (deletion of the short arm of chromosome 5), Down's syndrome, and neural tube defects.

Third-Trimester Amniocentesis.—The growth-retarded fetus is at increased risk for fetal distress and operative delivery. In view of the poor prognosis associated with many chromosomal malformations, it is important to attempt diagnosis prior to intervention in these pregnancies. Certainly, level II ultrasonography should be performed to detect anomalies such as neural tube defects and renal agenesis. Many of these defects are not compatible with extrauterine life, and diagnosis before delivery may be very important. In these cases, third-trimester amniocentesis to examine the chromosomes may alter management and allow the obstetrician to avoid operative intervention for a fetus that cannot survive the neonatal period. The consideration of third-trimester amniocentesis for karyotyping may be most important in cases of growth retardation when no clear cause may be found and in those cases where patterns of anomalies suggest a genetic basis for the impaired fetal growth (see Chapter 6).

PREMATURE RUPTURE OF MEMBRANES AND PREMATURITY

Recent studies have suggested that the growth-retarded fetus is at increased risk for premature rupture of the membranes (PROM) and premature delivery. Conversely, there is evidence that premature infants are more likely to exhibit some degree of impaired intrauterine growth. However, it is difficult to be certain that the premature infant is more likely to be growth retarded, because the growth curves at less than 37 weeks gestation are of questionable accuracy. These curves are necessarily based on the weights of infants born under nonphysiologic conditions such as premature labor, preterm PROM, or deteriorating maternal or fetal conditions. Because a preterm infant cannot be considered the product of a normal gestation, these growth curves may not be truly representative of normal growth and indeed may underestimate the expected intrauterine growth at a given gestation.

Recent improvement in sonographic estimation of fetal weight confirms the theory that pregnancies complicated by premature labor or PROM are more likely to result in the birth of a growth-retarded infant. Tamura et al.[32] reported that a significantly larger proportion of fetuses with subsequent premature delivery had sonographically determined biparietal diameter and abdominal circumference measurements below the 10th percentile at a comparable gestational age than did those "normal" fetuses who subsequently were delivered at term. Bottoms et al.[33] studied 397 pregnancies complicated by preterm PROM. Results indicated that the reduction in ultrasound measurements observed in pregnancies complicated by PROM was not due to mechanical effects, as previously believed, but reflected compromised intrauterine growth. These studies, although not conclusive, suggest a risk for premature delivery in the growth-retarded fetus. Further study is needed to examine the role of abnormal fetal growth in preterm delivery. It is interesting to postulate that premature labor or preterm PROM may represent yet another adaptation of the SGA fetus to a hostile intrauterine environment.

REFERENCES

1. Manara LR: Intrapartum fetal morbidity and mortality in intrauterine growth retarded infants. *J Am Osteopath Assoc* 1980; 80:101.
2. Morrison I, Olsen J: Weight-specific stillbirths and associated causes of death: An analysis of 765 stillbirths. *Am J Obstet Gynecol* 1985; 152:975.
3. Pitkin R: Fetal death: Diagnosis and management. *Am J Obstet Gynecol* 1987; 157:583.
4. Williams RL, Creasy RK, Cunningham GC, et al: Fetal growth and perinatal viability in California. *Obstet Gynecol* 1982; 59:624.
5. Tejani N, Mann LI, Weiss RR: Antenatal diagnosis and management of the small-for-gestational age fetus. *Obstet Gynecol* 1976; 47:31.
6. Usher RH: Clinical and therapeutic aspects of fetal malnutrition. *Pediatr Clin North Am* 1970; 17:169.
7. Gruenwald P: Chronic fetal distress and placental insufficiency. *Biol Neonate* 1963; 5:215.

8. Pose SV, Castello JB, Rojas-Mora EO, et al: Test of fetal tolerance to induced uterine contractions for the diagnosis of chronic distress, in *Perinatal Factors Affecting Human Development,* Pan-American Health Organization Scientific Publication No 185. Washington DC, World Health Organization, 1969, pp 96–104.
9. Lin CC, Devoe LD, River P, et al: Oxytocin challenge test and intrauterine growth retardation. *Am J Obstet Gynecol* 1981; 140:282.
10. Low JA, Pancham SR, Worthington D: Fetal heart deceleration patterns in relation to asphyxia and weight-gestational age percentile of the fetus. *Obstet Gynecol* 1976; 47:14.
11. Dawkins M: The small for dates baby. *Clin Dev Med* 1965; 19:33.
12. Second Report of British Perinatal Mortality Survey, in Butler NR, Alberman ED (eds): *Perinatal Problems.* Edinburgh, E & S Livingstone, 1969.
13. Lin CC, Moawad AH, Rosenow PJ, et al: Acid-base characteristics of fetuses with intrauterine growth retardation during labor and delivery. *Am J Obstet Gynecol* 1980; 137:553.
14. Bacsick RD: Meconium aspiration syndrome. *Pediatr Clin North Am* 1977; 24:642.
15. Carson BS, Losey RW, Bowes WA, et al: Combined obstetric and pediatric approach to prevent meconium aspiration syndrome. *Am J Obstet Gynecol* 1976; 126:712.
16. Gregory GA, Gooding CA, Phibbs RH, et al: Meconium aspiration in infants—A prospective study. *J Pediatr* 1974; 85:848.
17. Mitchell J, Schulman H, Fleischer A, et al: Meconium aspiration and fetal acidosis. *Obstet Gynecol* 1985; 65:352.
18. Brown BL, Gleicher N: Intrauterine meconium aspiration. *Obstet Gynecol* 1981; 57:26.
19. Dooley SL, Pesavento DJ, Depp R, et al: Meconium below the vocal cords at delivery: Correlation with intrapartum events. *Am J Obstet Gynecol* 1985; 153:767.
20. Davis RO, Philips JB, Harris BA, et al: Fetal meconium aspiration syndrome occurring despite airway management considered appropriate. *Am J Obstet Gynecol* 1985; 151:731.
21. Mann LI, Tejani NA, Weiss RR: Antenatal diagnosis and management of the small-for-gestational age fetus. *Am J Obstet Gynecol* 1974; 120:995.
22. Philipson EH, Sokol RJ, Williams T: Oligohydramnios: Clinical associations and predictive value for intrauterine growth retardation. *Am J Obstet Gynecol* 1983; 146:271.
23. Chamberlain PF, Manning FA, Morrison I, et al: Ultrasound evaluation of amniotic fluid volume. I. The relationship of marginal and decreased amniotic fluid volumes to perinatal outcome. *Am J Obstet Gynecol* 1984; 150:245.
24. Manning FA, Hall LM, Platt LD: Qualitative amniotic fluid volume determination by ultrasound: Antepartum detection of intrauterine growth retardation. *Am J Obstet Gynecol* 1981; 139:254.
25. Bastide A, Manning F, Harman C, et al: Ultrasound evaluation of amniotic fluid: Outcome of pregnancies with severe oligohydramnios. *Am J Obstet Gynecol* 1986; 154:895.

26. Barss VA, Benacerraf BR, Frigoletto FD: Second trimester oligohydramnios, a predictor of poor fetal outcome. *Obstet Gynecol* 1984; 64:608.
27. Dyer SN, Barton BK, Nelson LH: Elevated maternal serum alpha-fetoprotein levels in oligohydramnios: Poor prognosis for pregnancy outcome. *Am J Obstet Gynecol* 1987; 157:336.
28. Fantel AG, Shepard TH: Potter syndrome: Nonrenal features induced by oligoamnios. *Am J Dis Child* 1975; 129:1346.
29. Thibeault DW, Beatty EC, Hall RT, et al: Neonatal pulmonary hypoplasia with premature rupture of fetal membranes and oligohydramnios. *J Pediatr* 1985; 107:273.
30. Vintzileos AM, Campbell WA, Ingardia CJ, et al: The fetal biophysical profile and its predictive value. *Obstet Gynecol* 1983; 62:271.
31. Bottoms SF, Welch RA, Zador IE, et al: Limitations of using maximum vertical pocket and other sonographic evaluations of amniotic fluid volume to predict fetal growth: Technical or physiologic? *Am J Obstet Gynecol* 1986; 155:154.
32. Tamura RK, Sabbagha RE, Depp R, et al: Diminished growth in fetuses born preterm after spontaneous labor or rupture of membranes. *Am J Obstet Gynecol* 1984; 148:1105.
33. Bottoms SF, Welch RA, Zador IE, et al: Clinical interpretation of ultrasound measurements in preterm pregnancies with premature rupture of the membranes. *Obstet Gynecol* 1987; 69:358.

3

Neonatal Risks Associated With Intrauterine Growth Retardation

Nadya J. Kazzi, M.D.
Ronald L. Poland, M.D.

Intrauterine growth retardation (IUGR), an abnormality of fetal growth and development, affects 3% to 10% of all pregnancies. The incidence varies depending on the definition used to diagnose growth retardation. The most frequently used definition in the literature is birth weight less than the 10th percentile for gestational age. Other definitions include birth weight less than the 3rd, 5th, or 25th percentile, more than 2 SD below the mean, and ponderal index less than the 10th percentile.[1] It is important for the pediatrician to remember that the normative birth weight data derived from high-altitude populations, such as the Denver curves, cannot be used to diagnose IUGR in a sea level population because the two curves may differ by as much as 5 percentile points near term.[2] Such differences could result in significant underdiagnosis of IUGR.

Infants with IUGR represent a heterogenous group at risk for increased perinatal morbidity and mortality. The long-term morbidity in these infants depends on the cause of the growth retardation and the proper management of the immediate perinatal problems. The cause of IUGR is undetermined in up to 40% of cases. Most of these infants are constitutionally small and have a good outcome. In the remaining infants, growth retardation results from chronic progressive uteroplacental insufficiency secondary to maternal disease or to placental abnormalities; toxic exposures in utero, such as chronic alcohol exposure; intrauterine infections, particularly those occurring during

TABLE 3–1.
Comparison of the Incidence of Specific Problems Among Infants Admitted to a Tertiary Care Neonatal Unit: SGA vs AGA Infants

	SGA (n = 416)	AGA (n = 2,359)	Significance
Apgar score (mean ± SD)			
1 min	4.8 ± 2.6	6.1 ± 2.5	$P<0.01$
5 min	6.8 ± 2.2	7.6 ± 2.2	$P<0.01$
Apgar <6 (%)			
1 min	55.3	33.4	$P<0.01$
5 min	23.6	13.7	$P<0.01$
Meconium aspiration (%)	4.1	3.8	NS
Hypothermia (%)	6.0	2.4	$P<0.01$
Hypoglycemia (%)	7.2	6.8	NS
Polycythemia (%)	3.6	2.1	NS
Hypocalcemia (%)	9.1	5.5	$P<0.01$
Pulmonary hemorrhage (%)	5.3	2.3	$P<0.01$
Positive blood culture (%)	5.3	3.2	$P<0.05$

NS = not significant.

the first two trimesters of pregnancy; and some genetically determined conditions, including various chromosomal anomalies.

The most common perinatal complications encountered among infants with IUGR include perinatal asphyxia, meconium aspiration, hypothermia, hypoglycemia, polycythemia, hyperviscosity, hypocalcemia, pulmonary hemorrhage (rare), and depressed immune function. A comparison of the incidence of these various complications among IUGR infants at 25 to 40 weeks gestation as reported from the neonatal unit at Children's Hospital of Michigan is shown in Table 3–1. The increased awareness of the medical staff of the vulnerability of these infants during the perinatal period and the improvement in perinatal care have resulted in a decreased incidence of some complications in these infants.

In this chapter we discuss the pathophysiology of each of these complications. The perinatal management of IUGR is addressed in Chapters 12 and 13.

PERINATAL ASPHYXIA

Perinatal asphyxia is the most common cause of morbidity and mortality in infants with IUGR. Ninety percent of all asphyxial insults are noted during the antepartum and intrapartum periods. Many of these infants tolerate labor poorly, particularly those with growth retardation due to chronic uteroplacental insufficiency. In these infants the supply of fetal nutrients and transplacental oxygen transfer is already limited. Therefore any additional hypoxic stress during the delivery process may result in fetal hypoxia and acidosis. As many as one third of fetuses with IUGR demonstrate clinical signs of fetal distress during labor, including abnormal fetal heart rate patterns and fetal acidosis (pH <7.20) by fetal blood sampling.[3] There may be passage of meconium into the amniotic fluid, and the infant's Apgar score is frequently low. Depending on the timing and severity of the hypoxic-ischemic insult before adequate resuscitation occurs, multiple organ involvement may ensue, as summarized in Table 3–2. Most important among these is hypoxic-ischemic brain injury, the extent of which will determine the long-term neurologic morbidity in the infant.

Hypoxic-ischemic encephalopathy as described by Volpe[4] is a syndrome that develops in neonates a few hours after the perinatal insult. The infants are usually stuporous or comatose, with evidence of hypotonia and periodic breathing. Seizure activity is noted 6 to 12 hours after birth in 50% of these infants. The subsequent course is one of impaired consciousness and continuing seizures often unresponsive to anticonvulsant therapy. The long-term neurologic sequelae vary depending on areas of the brain most affected by the perinatal insult. Cortical neuronal necrosis in cerebellar and cerebral hemispheres results in mental retardation, seizures, and ataxia. Infarcts in the watershed areas and the periventricular regions manifest later as spastic quadriparesis and intellectual deficits, including various dyslectic syndromes and perceptual disturbances often apparent at school age. Severe mental impairment occurs only when the other motor defects are also severe. Finally necrosis of the thalamic and brain stem nuclei may result in choreoathetosis or spastic quadriparesis, with disturbances in thermoregulation and respiration. The prognosis in the neonate who sustains a hypoxic-ischemic insult varies according to the severity of the insult. Neurologic signs in the immediate neonatal period, such as seizures, hypotonia, or spasticity, carry a serious prognosis. In the premature infant the major complication of perinatal

TABLE 3–2.
Target Organs Involved in Perinatal Asphyxia

Organs	Condition
CNS	Brain edema; seizures, intracranial hemorrhage
Pulmonary	Meconium aspiration; persistent fetal circulation; respiratory distress syndrome
Cardiovascular	Hypotension and cardiac failure
Renal	Acute tubular neurosis; acute cortical nephron necrosis; oliguria and anuria with azotemia
Gastrointestinal	Necrotizing enterocolitis; stress ulcers; GI bleeding; hepatic injury with increase in AST, ALT, NH_3 levels; hyperbilirubinemia
Metabolic	Metabolic acidosis; hypoglycemia; hypocalcemia; hyperkalemia and hyponatremia; SIADH secretion
Hematologic	Disseminated intravascular coagulation; thrombocytopenia, neutropenia.

ALT = alanine aminotransferase; AST = aspartate aminotransferase; SIADH = syndrome of inappropriate secretion of antidiuretic hormone.

asphyxia is intraventricular hemorrhage, the extent of which mostly determines the neurologic outcome in these infants.

HYPOGLYCEMIA

Infants with IUGR are at a high risk for hypoglycemia (blood glucose less than 30 mg/dl). Lubchenco and Bard[5] have shown that the risk of hypoglycemia in newborn infants correlates best with the degree of maturation of the infant. They reported an incidence of hypoglycemia in 67% in preterm, 25% in term, and 18% in postterm IUGR infants. The hypoglycemia occurs mostly during the first few hours after birth, but can recur in the following 3 to 4 days of life. Infants whose growth in utero was compromised by chronic uteroplacental insufficiency or who sustained an episode of perinatal asphyxia are more likely to develop hypoglycemia.

The cause of hypoglycemia in these infants is multifactorial. Deficient hepatic and cardiac muscle glycogen stores result in decreased mobilization of glucose from these sites when needed in the immediate postnatal period. Hepatic gluconeogenesis is decreased because of limited ability to convert gluconeogenic substrates (e.g., alanine, lactate) present in adequate concentrations in the circulation. Diminished stores of body fat limit their ability to mobilize and oxidize free fatty acids and triglycerides. This oxidation normally provides the neonate with the energy needed for hepatic gluconeogenesis and spares the peripheral tissue utilization of glucose. Plasma levels of cortisol and growth hormone are elevated in the first few hours of life, indicating an intact pituitary-adrenal axis. Some investigators have reported deficient catecholamine release during periods of hypoglycemia in these infants.

Symptomatic hypoglycemia is a significant cause of morbidity and mortality, particularly in low birth weight and small for gestational age infants.[6] Glucose is the major metabolic fuel for the brain. Therefore it is not surprising that hypoglycemia causes signs of acute brain dysfunction such as apnea, jitteriness, lethargy, hypotonia, cyanosis, and convulsions. Glucose oxidation is also the major source of energy for the newborn heart where the alternative pathway for the degradation of fatty acids is also limited, particularly in infants with IUGR. As a result, prolonged untreated neonatal hypoglycemia can result in heart failure and eventually in cardiac arrest. The clinical manifestations of hypoglycemia may complicate other neonatal disorders, such as sepsis, intracranial hemorrhage, or congenital heart disease. Simple screening tests with chemical reagent strips (e.g., Dextrostix or Chemstrip BG) can be used at the bedside for early detection of hypoglycemia in infants at risk. These tests have been shown to correlate closely with laboratory blood glucose determinations. The Chemstrip has been shown to have a better correlation than the Dextrostix with blood glucose levels less than 40 mg/dl.

Animal and human neuropathologic studies showed evidence of wide-

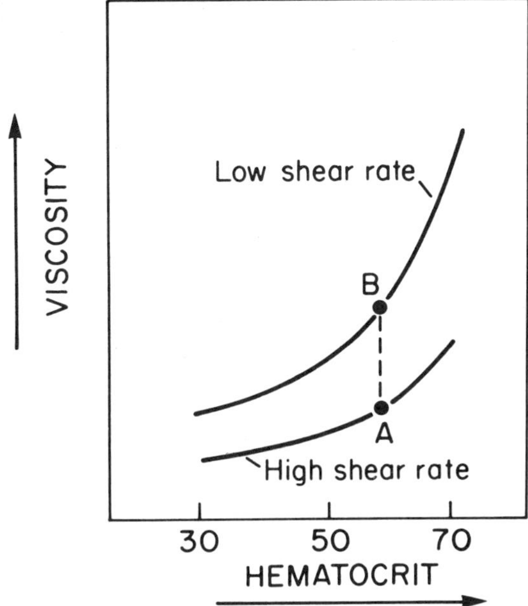

FIG 3–1.
Relationship between hematocrit and blood viscosity at high and low shear rates. (From Phibbs RH: Neonatal polycythemia, in Rudolph AM (ed): *Pediatrics,* ed 17. New York, Appleton-Century-Crofts, 1982. Used by permission.)

spread degeneration of neurons and injury to glial cells secondary to hypoglycemia.[7] As a result these infants may develop microcephaly, with dilated lateral ventricles secondary to a diminution in myelinated cerebral white matter. The vulnerability of the neonatal brain to hypoxic-ischemic injury is enhanced by a concomitant hypoglycemia. Therefore close monitoring of infants with IUGR postnatally for hypoglycemia and its prompt adequate therapy could significantly reduce neurologic long-term sequelae.

POLYCYTHEMIA AND HYPERVISCOSITY

The hyperviscosity syndrome is a symptom complex associated with decreased blood fluidity. Hyperviscosity and polycythemia are not synonymous; not all polycythemic neonates have hyperviscous blood, and vice versa. Blood viscosity in general is determined by three major components: the concentration of cellular elements including red blood cells, white blood cells, and platelets; the concentrations of plasma elements such as plasma proteins (e.g., fibrinogen, immunoglobulins) and chylomicrons; and the deformability of the red cell. Of these factors the red cell mass, or hematocrit, is the most important in determining the blood viscosity in the neonatal period. The relationship between hematocrit and blood viscosity is shown in Figure 3–1. When hematocrit is less than 60% to 65% the relationship is almost linear.

At higher hematocrit values it becomes exponential. The plasma viscosity in the newborn period is identical to that in adults. Neonatal red cells are, however, less deformable than those in adults. Their deformability is further reduced by hypoxia and acidosis, both of which occur with perinatal asphyxia. Therefore infants with IUGR may be at greater risk for developing clinical manifestations of hyperviscosity.

Hyperviscosity secondary to polycythemia is common in infants with IUGR, with an incidence of 15% to 17% compared with 4% in infants appropriate for gestational age (AGA).[8] It appears to be more frequent among infants with growth retardation secondary to placental abnormalities or to maternal disease. The cause of polycythemia in these infants is multifactorial. Chronic fetal hypoxia is thought to be the main stimulus for enhanced erythropoietin secretion and increased red cell mass production. In addition, with perinatal asphyxia there is evidence in animals and in humans of placental fetal transfusion to maintain oxygen supply to the fetus.[9] Finally, delay in cord clamping at delivery may increase the neonatal blood volume by as much as 80 to 100 ml, increasing further the red cell mass of the newborn infant.

Virtually all clinical manifestations of polycythemia are due to the associated increase in blood viscosity. Sludging of the blood flow occurs in various organs including the central nervous system, lungs, heart, gastrointestinal tract, and kidneys. The infant manifests varying degrees of plethora, cyanosis, and jitteriness. As the severity of the polycythemia increases there is evidence of respiratory distress, congestive heart failure, seizures, and even intracranial bleeding secondary to thrombotic disease. Other complications include hypoglycemia, hyperbilirubinemia, thrombocytopenia, renal vein thrombosis, and gangrene of any of the extremities. Hyperviscosity is a cause for increased short- and long-term morbidity in infants with IUGR and adequate screening for hyperviscosity is recommended. Measurement of whole blood viscosity is not routinely available in clinical situations. A central venous hematocrit value of 65% or greater is generally accepted for the diagnosis of polycythemia and hyperviscosity because those hematocrit values are associated with a viscosity value greater than 2 SD above the normal mean for term infants.[8, 10]

HYPOTHERMIA

Infants with IUGR are at risk for excessive heat loss in the immediate neonatal period. Immediately after birth, and on exposure to a cold environment, the newborn infant attempts to maintain a stable body temperature by two major mechanisms: increasing endogenous heat production and limiting the dissipation of heat to the environment.[11] Brown adipose tissue is the main site for thermogenesis in the newborn infant. These stores are not depleted in infants with IUGR; however, hypoxia and probably hypoglycemia could interfere with heat production in this tissue. The lack of an adequately developed insulating layer of adipose tissue and the large body surface area compared with that in normally grown infants limit the ability of infants with IUGR to prevent heat loss from the body when exposed to a cold stress. Therefore particular attention in keeping these infants warm postnatally is recommended, especially if perinatal asphyxia warrants resuscitation in the delivery room.

MECONIUM ASPIRATION

Meconium staining of the amniotic fluid occurs in 8% to 10% of all deliveries. The passage of meconium in utero has been attributed to hypoxia causing increased peristalsis in the fetal gut and sphincter relaxation. It is considered a sign of fetal distress only when accompanied by abnormal fetal heart rate patterns or evidence of fetal acidosis on fetal scalp blood sampling.[12] Active intervention for immediate delivery may be necessary in such circumstances, particularly in postterm and infants with IUGR, because they are at increased risk for meconium aspiration in the peripartum period. If meconium aspiration occurs, the infant will manifest various degrees of respiratory distress, tachypnea, cyanosis with evidence of hypoxemia, and mixed acidosis on arterial blood sampling. The respiratory distress in these infants is attributed to the partial blocking of the distal airways by meconium, resulting in areas of atelectasis or overdistended alveoli secondary to a ball valve effect. Such alveoli may rupture, causing air to leak into the pleural space, interstitium, or pericardium, further compromising pulmonary and myocardial functions. Persistent fetal circulation and pulmonary hypertension often accompany meconium aspiration, particularly in infants with evidence of prolonged intrauterine hypoxia, such as postterm and IUGR infants. Although meconium aspiration can occur in utero, it doesn't occur frequently. Therefore immediate proper suctioning of the oropharynx and trachea of these infants in the delivery room is necessary and has been shown to reduce mortality and morbidity significantly.[13]

HYPOCALCEMIA

Serum calcium concentrations in the neonate during the first 3 days of life correlate with gestational age more than with birth weight. Thus infants with IUGR appear at no greater risk for hypocalcemia than do AGA infants. However, growth-retarded infants who sustain an episode of perinatal asphyxia and require alkali therapy to correct metabolic acidosis may have a higher incidence of neonatal hypocalcemia.[14] Correction of hypocalcemia often is spontaneous.

IMMUNE FUNCTION

Protein caloric malnutrition in postnatal life results in a profound decrease in cellular immunity. With dietary treatment, however, the immune function can be restored within weeks. Infants with IUGR have evidence of impaired cell-mediated immunity, a low number of B-lymphocytes, and decreased concentrations of immunoglobulins. These changes, however, seem to persist throughout early childhood.[15] Antibody responses after immunization have been reported to be lower than in AGA infants. As a result, infants with IUGR are thought to be at a greater risk for infection. Chandra[16] reported a higher incidence of upper and lower respiratory tract infections among infants with IUGR compared with AGA infants, similar to the incidence in other infants with a defect in immune function. Infants with IUGR are at risk for infections with opportunistic organisms such as *Pneumocystis carinii.*

REFERENCES

1. Seeds JW: Impaired fetal growth—Definition and clinical diagnosis. *Obstet Gynecol* 1984; 64:303.
2. Williams RL: Fetal growth and perinatal viability in California. *Obstet Gynecol* 1982; 59:624.
3. Low JA, Boston RW, Pancham SR: Fetal asphyxia during the intrapartum period in intrauterine growth retarded infants. *Am J Obstet Gynecol* 1972; 113:351.
4. Volpe JJ: Hypoxic-ischemic encephalopathy: Neuropathology and clinical aspects, in Volpe JJ (ed): *Neurology of the Newborn.* Philadelphia, WB Saunders Co, 1981, pp 180–238.
5. Lubchenco LO, Bard H: Incidence of hypoglycemia in newborn infants classified by birth weight and gestational age. *Pediatrics* 1971; 47:831.
6. Beard A, Cornblath M, Gentz J, et al: Neonatal hypoglycemia: A discussion. *J Pediatr* 1971; 79:314.
7. Bankers BQ: The neuropathological effects of anoxia and hypoglycemia in the newborn. *Dev Med Child Neurol* 1967; 9:544.
8. Hakanson DO, Oh W: Hyperviscosity in the small for gestational infants. *Biol Neonate* 1980; 37:109.
9. Oh W, Omori O, Emmanouilides GC, et al: Placenta to lamb fetus transfusion in utero during acute hypoxia. *Am J Obstet Gynecol* 1975; 122:316.
10. Gross GP, Hathaway WE, McCaughey HR: Hyperviscosity in the neonate. *J Pediatr* 1973; 82:1004.
11. Sinclair JC: *Metabolic Rate and Temperature Control.* Springfield, Ill, Charles C Thomas, Publisher, 1976, pp 354–415.
12. Miller FC, Sacks DA, Szeya Y, et al: Significance of meconium during labor. *Am J Obstet Gynecol* 1975; 122:573.
13. Gregory GA, Gooding CA, Phibbs RH, et al: Meconium aspiration in infants—A prospective study. *J Pediatr* 1974; 85:848.
14. Tsang RC, Gigger M, Oh W, et al: Studies in calcium metabolism in infants with intrauterine growth retardation. *J Pediatr* 1975; 86:936.

15. Chandra RK: Fetal malnutrition and postnatal immunocompetence. *Am J Dis Child* 1975; 129:450.
16. Chandra RK: Nutrition, immunity, and infection: Present knowledge and future directions. *Lancet* 1983; 1:688.

4

Developmental Sequelae Following Intrauterine Growth Retardation

Vincent L. Smeriglio, Ph.D.

This chapter focuses on developmental outcomes following intrauterine growth retardation (IUGR). First an overview of developmental outcomes for full-term and preterm infants with IUGR is provided. Then attention is focused on development within subgroups of the IUGR population designated by timing of the intrauterine insult, by maternal conditions during pregnancy, and by neonatal medical conditions. For each of these three subgroups a Highlights and Commentary section is followed by a more in-depth presentation of available information. In the last part of the chapter the importance of associated medical conditions and of the postnatal environment of the IUGR infant and child is discussed.

To provide a perspective on the sources of the developmental outcome information, a brief characterization of IUGR developmental follow-up investigations is included in these introductory paragraphs. These comments focus on IUGR definitions, birth weight for gestational age standards, types of developmental outcomes utilized, changing IUGR populations, sample exclusions, and losses to follow-up.

As in other areas of IUGR investigation, in developmental follow-up studies the specific percentile birth weight for gestational age used to define IUGR has varied, often being the 10th percentile and sometimes the 5th, the 3rd, or the 25th percentile. IUGR has also been defined as birth weight 2 SD below the mean for gestational age.

A number of published birth weight for gestational age standards have been used in studies of developmental outcomes, and several of these are identified in discussions later in the chapter. Some investigators have used their own study populations as the basis for standards of percentile for gestational age.

The most frequently seen outcomes in reports of developmental follow-up of IUGR are results of infant development tests, performance on intelligence tests, and occurrence of disabilities (physical and mental). Several authors[1–3] have commented on problems in the reporting of handicapping conditions, including the issue of distinction between the terms disability and handicap. The potential value of more attention to behavioral outcomes has been noted in the literature.[4]

A variety of developmental and intelligence tests have been used, and the definition of disability has been variable. The limited predictability of developmental test performance in the first 2 years of life[5] limits the usefulness of information from those study subjects not followed up beyond 2 years of age. This predictability issue may be somewhat less of a problem for those infants with very low performance[5] and for very low birth weight preterm infants,[6] especially if tested after 14 months of age.[7]

Continuing changes in survival, physical condition, and health status of children with IUGR have important implications for developmental projections based on current knowledge. Two additional factors with implications for generalizability of available findings are exclusions from study samples and losses to follow-up. Several investigators have excluded certain infants with IUGR from study, often based on methodologic considerations. For example, those infants with a history of intrauterine infection or evidence of congenital anomalies or chromosomal abnormalities frequently have been excluded. Those surviving study subjects who participate in follow-up evaluations may differ in important ways from those who do not participate.

The complexity of determining developmental sequelae of IUGR is well recognized. IUGR and the subsequent development of the infant occur in a context of many related factors, including maternal conditions, family conditions, neonatal medical conditions, and postnatal environment and experiences. Some of these factors themselves have been shown to be related to child development. Figure 4–1 illustrates some of the interrelationships that are important to consider when attempting to determine associations between IUGR and later development.

The particular combination of related factors varies across the population of infants with IUGR, making them a very heterogeneous group. This heterogeneity may help in interpretation of conflicting findings in different investigations, and should also confirm the clinician's interest in looking beyond the IUGR classification when evaluating later development.

Throughout this chapter the terms "IUGR," "small for gestational age" (SGA), "small for dates" (SFD), and "light for dates" (LFD) are used interchangeably, but IUGR is emphasized. Further emphasis is placed on studies that explicitly identify IUGR (SGA, SFD, LFD) study groups. Although follow-

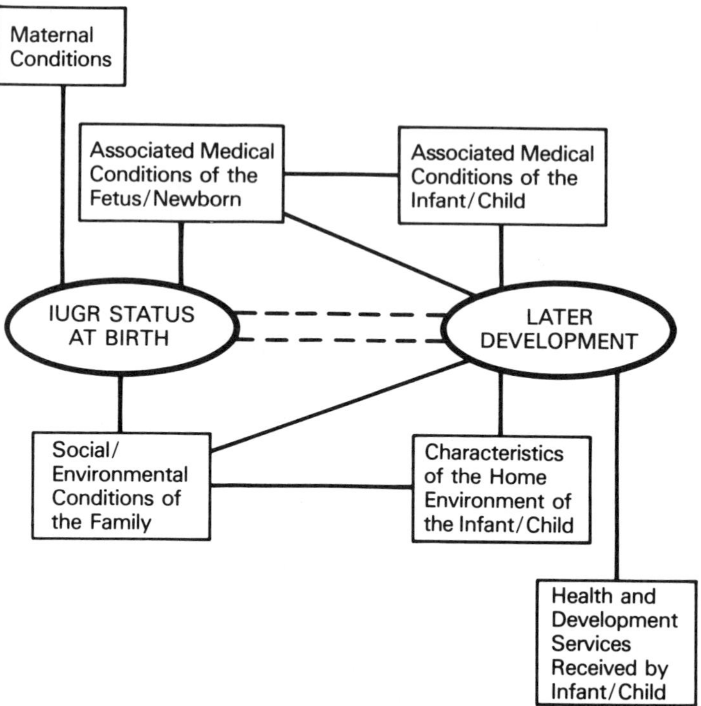

FIG 4–1.
Interrelationships among factors associated with intrauterine growth retardation and later development.

up studies of low birth weight (and especially very low birth weight) infants are likely to include IUGR infants in their samples, from reports of those investigations it is often not possible to identify these infants as a separate group. The emphasis on investigations that explicitly identify IUGR study groups is not meant to diminish the value of birth weight as an important variable. Relationships between birth weight (without consideration of gestational age) and child development have been documented repeatedly.[8–10] As will be shown, some investigators have documented that within the IUGR population birth weight is an important factor relative to later development. In addition, SGA versus appropriate for gestational age (AGA) comparisons may differentiate development more within some birth weight categories than within others.[11]

OVERVIEW OF DEVELOPMENTAL OUTCOMES FOLLOWING IUGR

As noted by several authors,[2, 12–16] IUGR developmental follow-up findings across investigations have been diverse and sometimes conflicting. Nonetheless, it has been possible for those reviewing work in the field to draw some general conclusions. Investigations focused on full-term infants with IUGR have been more numerous, have included a wider range of outcomes, and have followed development for longer periods than has been the case in studies focused on preterm infants with IUGR.

Follow-Up of Full-Term Infants With IUGR

In her comprehensive review of studies, Allen[2] concluded the following about developmental outcomes of full-term SGA infants.

1. The vast majority of full-term SGA infants demonstrate normal intelligence on tests administered in the preschool and school years. The mean IQ of the SGA population often has been somewhat lower than that of comparison groups, but the difference seldom has been statistically significant.
2. The vast majority of full-term SGA infants do not show evidence of major handicap on follow-up, although there is some suggestion of a slightly increased risk for cerebral palsy and mental retardation in this population in comparison with AGA infants.
3. There is evidence of an increased risk in full-term SGA infants for minimal cerebral dysfunction, including increased incidence of speech and language problems, minor neurologic findings, attention deficits, and school failures despite normal intelligence.

As noted, various definitions of IUGR have been used in studies of developmental follow-up, including less than the 10th percentile and less than the 5th percentile birth weight for gestational age. In the longitudinal study of Neligan et al.[17] the full-term (i.e., ≥255 days, or 36 weeks) IUGR sample was subdivided into those infants with birth weight between the 5th and 10th percentiles for gestational age (rather light for dates, or RLFD) and those infants with birth weight below the 5th percentile for gestational age (very light for dates, or VLFD). The study included numerous developmental outcomes measured at 5, 6, or 7 years of age (e.g., intelligence tests, neurologic assessments, language development tests, behavioral and temperament measures). The VLFD group more often performed significantly less well relative to a randomly drawn comparison group than did the RLFD group. Therefore birth weight within this full-term IUGR group was a factor of significance relative to developmental outcomes. This is especially interesting in that in this sample even the VLFD infants did not have very low birth weights (mean 2397 gm). These findings support the concept that the particular birth weight for gestational age used to define IUGR may well be of importance regarding the developmental outcome to be expected.

Follow-Up of Preterm Infants With IUGR

Conclusions regarding developmental outcomes in preterm infants with IUGR are of necessity still limited and tentative. This is a reflection of the extent of information available and the sometimes conflicting findings reported. Previous authors have noted that sample sizes have been small,[2, 18] comparison groups have differed across studies,[2] and virtually no information about development at school age has been reported.[2] Furthermore, the heterogeneity of the preterm IUGR population is likely to contribute to different findings across samples. This heterogeneity itself is likely to shift with changes in the survival patterns in the preterm, very low birth weight population. The majority of recent reports on development in preterm infants with IUGR provides information on babies born between 1974 and 1976.[12, 18–23] Other factors possibly contributing to differences in findings across studies include variation in the proportion of inborn infants versus outborn transfers in the samples, variation in obstetric practices, and variation in definition of handicaps.

After review and analysis of reports of developmental outcomes in the preterm IUGR population, Allen[2] reached the following conclusions:

1. Preterm SGA infants appear to have a higher incidence of major handicap than the general population does.
2. Preterm SGA infants probably have a higher incidence of major handicap than term SGA infants do.
3. Preterm SGA infants perhaps have a higher incidence of major handicap than preterm AGA infants do.

The limited and tentative nature of the above conclusions emphasizes the need for additional investigations of the developmental outcomes of preterm infants with IUGR. Furthermore, the importance of longer follow-up of developmental functioning is highlighted by the findings of Vohr and Oh,[21] though caution in interpretation must be exercised given the small sample size of that study. Compared with AGA preterm infants, SGA preterm infants had significantly lower developmental test performance at 9 months and at 1 and 2 years of age and significantly lower IQ scores at 3 years. At 4 and 5 years of age, however, there was no statistical difference between the groups on IQ test performance. One of the 19 SGA preterm infants tested at 5 years of age had an IQ below 80, compared with none of the 16 AGA preterm infants.

Summary

Allen[2] noted that although the SGA concept has served a useful purpose and continues to be used to identify a population of newborn infants in need of closer examination, the SGA classification has also led to confusion about developmental outcome. She and others[13, 14] have emphasized the need to separate the heterogeneous IUGR population into more homogeneous subgroups, potentially to establish a better understanding of the development of infants with IUGR and therefore more accurate prognoses and more appropriate plans for postnatal services.

DEVELOPMENTAL FOLLOW-UP OF IUGR SUBGROUPS

The specific basis used for subdividing the IUGR population has differed considerably across investigations, and some methodologic limitations exist in this work. Nonetheless, these investigations represent important efforts toward reducing IUGR heterogeneity. Several representative studies are discussed in each of three areas that have served as the basis for subgroup formation: timing of the prenatal insult, maternal conditions during pregnancy, and neonatal medical conditions.

Timing of Prenatal Insult

Highlights and Commentary.—To estimate the timing of prenatal insult, investigators have used serial ultrasonic cephalometry[24–27] during pregnancy and ponderal index [(Weight/Length^3) $\times$ 100] values in the neonatal period.[14, 28] Published work on timing has been done in full-term infants with IUGR. Several developmental measures and follow-up ages have been included in the published reports. Similarities were found among children from three different populations (a sample in England in which ultrasound was used[24–27] and samples from Guatemala[14] and the Netherlands[28] using ponderal index). Based on these results from ponderal index and ultrasound studies, Villar et al.[14] suggested a time-effect relationship between timing of intrauterine insult and later developmental performance. The IUGR groups presumed to have experienced early insult (those whose head growth slowed before 26 weeks gestation as demonstrated by ultrasound and those whose ponderal index suggested proportionate insult in both weight and length) consistently demonstrated the lowest developmental performance. Those infants who presumably experienced late insult (those whose head growth slowed after 26 weeks gestation and those whose ponderal index suggested disproportionate insult in weight growth) usually demonstrated developmental performance levels between those of the early-insult and appropriate for dates (AFD) comparison groups.

Timing by Ultrasonic Cephalometry.—A series of publications[24–27] reported on a group of infants in England whose development was followed to ages 28 months to 9 years. Infants classified as SGA or SFD were those whose birth weight was below the 10th percentile for gestational age by the Tanner and Thomson[29] standards. All infants were born at 37 or more completed weeks of gestation. Beginning prior to 30 weeks gestation and continuing to within 2 weeks of delivery, serial ultrasonic measurements of the biparietal diameter were conducted using the method reported by Campbell.[30] Onset of slow head growth was taken to be when the weekly increment in biparietal diameter fell below the 5th percentile (relative to normal biparietal diameter curves[31]) over 2 weeks or more.

Three IUGR subgroups were formed on the basis of onset of slow head growth: at or before 26 weeks gestation, between 27 and 34 weeks gestation, and after 34 weeks gestation; a fourth subgroup of infants with IUGR had no evidence of slow intrauterine head growth. The distribution of social classes using a classification system based on father's occupation was reported as not significantly different between the four subgroups.[24] It was also reported that there were no differences between the groups in incidence of birth asphyxia, serum bilirubin concentration, respiratory problems, minor congenital defects, neonatal or later convulsions, major infections of the newborn, maternal age or parity, incidence of preeclamptic toxemia, or hypertension in the pregnancy.

Developmental outcomes for these infants with IUGR have been reported for mean ages of 4 years,[24] 5.1 years,[25,27] and 7.2 years.[26] Fifty-seven infants were assessed at mean age 4 years (range 28 to 84 months), 51 at mean age 5.1 years (range 3 to 7 years), and 45 at mean age 7.2 years (range 5 to 9 years). The specific groups compared have varied somewhat across reports, but a frequent comparison has been made between the group whose head growth slowed at or before 26 weeks gestation (early onset) and all other infants with IUGR in the sample (i.e., slowed head growth after 26 weeks gestation or no evidence of slowed intrauterine head growth).

On developmental test performance at ages 4 and 5.1 years, mean scores on overall developmental indices were significantly lower for the group with early-onset IUGR relative to the combined late-onset/no slowing IUGR group. These mean scores for both groups were within what appears to be a normal range. When compared with appropriate for dates (AFD) matched control subjects at mean age 5.1 years, children with early-onset IUGR showed significantly lower developmental performance, but the combined late-onset/no slowing group showed comparable performance. The control subjects were individually matched with the children with IUGR for sex, social class, birth order, and birth date within 6 months.

Scores on several subscales were also significantly lower for the early-onset group in comparison with the late-onset/no slowing group at 4 years (eye and hand coordination, motor development, practical reasoning, and personal-social subscales) and at 5.1 years (perceptual-performance, quantitative, and motor subscales). The investigators[27] pointed out that a major contribution to the difference at 5.1 years of age between the early-onset group and their AFD controls on the overall developmental score was the lower performance of the early-onset group on the perceptual-performance subscale, which measures ability to understand and carry out instructions and to copy and classify shapes.

While acknowledging the impossibility of knowing what caused the poorer developmental performance in the early-onset group, the authors speculated that it may be related to growth retardation during vital periods of brain development.[27] They noted that there is a period of rapid brain growth from mid-gestation through the second year of postnatal life, that neuronal multiplication in the forebrain occurs between 10 and 18 weeks of gestation, and that glial cell multiplication begins immediately thereafter. Consequently they presented the possibility that retardation of brain growth during the second trimester may affect both cerebral and cerebellar development.

Information pertaining to achievement and behavior in school has been reported for these children at mean age 7.2 years.[26] Teachers rated each child relative to other children of the same age in the class in 10 different areas of schoolwork and assessed the child's behavior in 16 specific areas.

Included in the investigators' summary of their findings were the following suggestions:

1. Among those children with IUGR studied, the most likely to have poor school achievement and behavioral problems were boys in whom head growth slowed before 34 weeks gestation.
2. Both the boys and the girls in whom head growth slowed before 34 weeks were thought to exhibit more extreme behavior than the other children with IUGR or their AFD comparisons.
3. There were sex differences in the extreme behavioral patterns in the group with slowed head growth before 34 weeks: the boys tended to be clumsy, worried, fidgety, not very adaptable, and unable to concentrate, whereas the girls tended to cry more often, bully other children, and be irritable.
4. Both boys and girls in the group with slowed head growth before 26 weeks had problems with reading, writing, drawing, and concentrating, but the girls had less difficulty with schoolwork than did the boys.

The investigators pointed out the importance of both sex and social class relative to later development in infants with IUGR.

In summary, for these children with IUGR the timing of the prenatal insult as measured by ultrasonic cephalometry appeared to be related to performance and behavior in school and to developmental test performance. Although information on intrauterine timing of slowed head growth in combination with IUGR diagnosis at birth was useful in prediction of later developmental functioning, this is not to say that prenatal ultrasonic measurement of head growth detected the IUGR or predicted developmental outcome independently of the IUGR diagnosis at birth. Difficulties in the prenatal detection of IUGR, particularly early in pregnancy, have been pointed out by other authors.[32–34]

Timing Based on Ponderal Index.—Ponderal index values have been used to infer timing of prenatal insult in infants with IUGR based on the following reasoning. Peak velocity of fetal length growth occurs during the second trimester of pregnancy, and peak velocity of fetal weight growth in the third trimester.[35] Consequently, if a fetus experiences chronic intrauterine retardation from early in the pregnancy, the newborn may be growth retarded (IUGR), with proportionately affected weight and length. The fetus experiencing a more acute intrauterine insult later in the pregnancy may also be growth retarded (IUGR), with disproportionately affected weight. Those infants with proportionately affected weight and length, although presumed to have experienced chronic intrauterine insult, have normal or adequate ponderal index values (IUGR-API), and their IUGR has sometimes been referred to as proportioned, symmetric, or "nonwasted." Those infants with disproportionate weight growth, presumed to have experienced acute intrauterine insult late in pregnancy, have low ponderal index values (IUGR-LPI), with IUGR sometimes called disproportioned, asymmetric, or "wasted."

Developmental outcomes have been reported for a group of rural Guatemalan infants with IUGR divided into subgroups based on ponderal index in the newborn period.[14] All infants in this report were born at 37 or more weeks gestation and were without serious neonatal illness or congenital malformations. Infants with IUGR were those with birth weight for gestational age below the 10th percentile using the standards published by Hoffman et al.[36] An AFD (birth weight for gestational age between the 10th and 90th percentiles) comparison group was also part of the study. The infants with IUGR were subdivided into two groups: IUGR-LPI and IUGR-API, respectively, if below or above the 10th percentile of ponderal index for gestational age using the standards of Lubchenco et al.[37] In the newborn period there were 21 IUGR-LPI infants, 38 IUGR-API infants, and 146 AFD comparison infants.

Infant developmental test performance was assessed at 6, 15, and 24 months using the Composite Infant Scale, which measures mental and motor functioning. At 3 years of age a battery of developmental tests was administered to assess reasoning, verbal processes, learning, perceptual analytic skills, and memory. In examining developmental performance the investigators statistically controlled for sex of the child, socioeconomic status, morbidity, and nutritional supplementation. At 6 and 15 months no significant differences in developmental performance were found among the three groups (IUGR-API, IUGR-LPI, and AFD comparison infants). At 24 months the IUGR-API group had a significantly lower mental performance score than did the AFD comparison infants when there was control for level of stimulation in the home and for a composite maternal index reflecting the mother's vocabulary, years of school completed, and "modernity" (e.g., reading of newspapers, travel, and knowledge of current events). The IUGR-LPI group was not significantly different from the AFD comparison group at 24 months.

At 3 years of age a pattern emerged in which the AFD group had the highest scores on a variety of tests, the IUGR-API group the lowest scores, and the IUGR-LPI group had intermediate performance. On the cognitive composite score, similar to overall IQ, the AFD group showed a mean score at the 63rd percentile. Each of the two IUGR groups had a significantly lower mean score relative to the AFD group. Again the children in the IUGR-API group were at the lowest level (38th percentile) and the IUGR-LPI children at the intermediate level (48th percentile).

Therefore, although the IUGR-API group appeared to be at greater developmental risk than the IUGR-LPI group, the IUGR-LPI group did seem to be at some developmental risk. This concept of some developmental risk among IUGR-LPI infants is supported by the findings of an investigation comparing IUGR-LPI and AFD children in the Netherlands.[28] On developmental follow-up at mean age 3 years 2 months (range 31 to 42 months), the IUGR-LPI group scored lower than the AFD group on several measures of behavioral and neurologic functioning, although not always to a statistically significant degree.

Maternal Conditions During Pregnancy

Highlights and Commentary.—Development following IUGR has been studied in relation to maternal hypertension, placental function estimates (urinary estriol, serum cystine aminopeptidase, and human chorionic somatomammotropin), antepartum hemorrhage, and composite indices of maternal conditions. Conclusions are still very limited. Findings are sometimes inconsistent, as in the case of hypertensive disorders.[13, 15] Sometimes only short follow-up periods have been reported, as in the case of placental function estimates.[38, 39] Antepartum hemorrhage[17] and composite maternal conditions indices[9] have been found to have relatively little association with measures of childhood developmental functioning. Comparisons of findings across investigations are complicated by variation in measures used to define the specific maternal conditions, definition of IUGR, methods of statistical analysis, proportion of preterm and full-term infants in the sample (sometimes not specified), and other population characteristics.

Hypertensive Disorders.—One study[13] reported findings in two groups of children with IUGR: 20 whose mothers had acute or chronic hypertensive disorders (as defined by the American College of Obstetricians and Gynecologists) during pregnancy and 35 whose mothers did not have hypertensive disease during pregnancy. IUGR status was defined by birth weight for gestational age less than the 10th percentile using the Lubchenco standards. Developmental assessments were conducted between 4 and 7 years of age.

Performance on several measures reflecting intellectual functioning, perceptual-motor functioning, and achievement (arithmetic and reading) typically was higher for children whose mothers had hypertension, although only for one measure (verbal IQ) was the difference statistically significant when socioeconomic status was controlled. In contrast, of the five major neurologic abnormalities seen for the entire group, three were in children whose mothers had hypertension during pregnancy, leading the investigators to suggest that infants of these mothers are unusually susceptible to the effects of hypoxia in the intrapartum period and that careful monitoring during labor is mandatory.

In another investigation examining subgroups of infants with IUGR based on presence or absence of maternal hypertension and preeclampsia,[15] no differences were found between groups on developmental performance at 4 years. The mostly full-term IUGR group had birth weight more than 2 SD below the mean for gestational age as defined by the British Perinatal Mortality Survey.[40] Developmental functioning was assessed in five areas: gross motor, fine motor, visuomotor, language, and comprehension. Hypertension was defined as blood pressure 140/90 mm Hg or higher recorded at any time during pregnancy. Diagnosis of moderate or severe preeclampsia required definite albuminuria on at least two occasions. All of the women with moderate or severe preeclampsia also had hypertension. Those women with mild preeclampsia were included in the normotensive nonpreeclamptic group.[41]

The reasons for the different findings regarding the relationship between maternal hypertension and developmental performance in these two studies[13, 15] are not clear. Possibilities include the differences between the studies in population characteristics, postnatal environments, definitions of hypertension, developmental outcome measures, statistical procedures and significance levels, and timing of delivery in the groups with hypertension.

Other Maternal Conditions During Pregnancy.—In two longer follow-up studies[9, 17] using multiple regression techniques to examine a large number of potential predictors of developmental outcome of infants with IUGR, measures of maternal conditions during pregnancy were found to be relatively weak predictors. In full-term VLFD infants (at or below the 5th percentile for gestational age), antepartum hemorrhage showed limited association with a wide range of measures of developmental functioning at 5, 6, or 7 years of age.[17] Similarly, neither a maternal delivery complications index nor a medical conditions of pregnancy index (sum of conditions of preeclamptic toxemia, hemorrhage, and cervical incompetence experienced during the pregnancy) nor a general medical conditions of pregnancy index was found to be a strong predictor of intelligence test performance at 10 years of age in a mixed group of preterm and full-term infants with IUGR (birth weight at or below the 10th percentile for gestational age).[9]

Neonatal Medical Conditions

Highlights and Commentary.— Conclusions are very limited for reduction of IUGR heterogeneity on the basis of neonatal medical conditions and complications. In addition to some of the typical methodologic limitations (e.g., variation in definitions of IUGR and of medical conditions), investigations in this area are particularly limited by restricted sample sizes and frequent absence of statistical testing. Several specific neonatal conditions and complications have been represented in the investigations,[9, 15, 17, 18, 42, 43] a frequent one being asphyxia. Both full-term and preterm infants with IUGR have been studied. Results have shown some inconsistencies across investigations.

Asphyxia.—The particular focus of one investigation was nonasphyxiated full-term SGA infants.[42] Intelligence testing was carried out when the children were at a mean age of 16.5 years (range 13 to 19 years). The authors mentioned a comparison of these 33 children with 11 asphyxiated SGA children (presumed tested at comparable age). Five of the asphyxiated SGA children had 5–minute Apgar scores ≤5, and six had Apgar scores ≤5 at 1 minute but >5 at 5 minutes. No statistical comparison was reported, but for the nonasphyxiated group the mean overall IQ was 101, and for the asphyxiated group 87.1. In this sample of SGA infants birth weight was more than 2 SD below the mean on the Usher and McLean standards.[44] The children were born between 1960 and 1966.

Commey and Fitzhardinge,[18] observed development during the first 2 years of life in preterm (<37 weeks gestation) infants with birth weights more than 2 SD below the mean on the Usher and McLean standards.[44] All infants were outborn and were admitted to a regional neonatal intensive care unit (NICU) within hours of delivery. Birth asphyxia was defined as a 5–minute Apgar score <6 or need for positive-pressure resuscitation for longer than 2 minutes. In addition to birth asphyxia, several other neonatal complications (CNS depression on admission, mechanical ventilation, respiratory distress syndrome, primary or late apnea, seizures, intracranial hemorrhage, meningitis, hyperbilirubinemia requiring exchange transfusion, and necrotizing enterocolitis) were examined in relation to developmental outcomes. The authors reported that the only statistically significant association shown was that between later handicap and the presence of cerebral depression on NICU admission, but they noted that birth asphyxia was an earlier complication in 21 of 24 surviving infants admitted with cerebral depression.

Within a group of infants with IUGR examined for developmental functioning (gross motor, fine motor, visuomotor, language, comprehension) at 4 years of age, asphyxia at birth ("regular respiration not established within 5 minutes"[45]) was not associated with developmental outcome.[15] The vast majority of infants in this IUGR group were born at term. IUGR status was defined as birth weight more than 2 SD below the mean for gestational age using the British Perinatal Mortality Survey.[40] Injury at birth, fetal distress, and other neonatal problems also were reported as not statistically related to developmental outcome at 4 years of age. In a group of full-term infants whose birth weight for gestational age was at or below the 5th percentile, delay in establishing regular respiration (1 minute, 1 to 4 minutes, or more than 5 minutes) was statistically predictive of developmental outcomes measured at 6 and 7 years of age.[17]

Other Neonatal Conditions.—Westwood et al.[42] identified four subgroups within a sample of nonasphyxiated full-term SGA children: those with neonatal hypoglycemia (serum glucose 20 mg/dl at least once during the first 24 hours), those with neonatal polycythemia (hematocrit 65% at least once during the hospital stay), those with birth length below the 3rd percentile, and those with both birth length and head circumference below the 3rd percentile. No data or statistics were provided, but the investigators reported that none of the subgroups had lower cognitive scores (at mean age 16.5 years) when compared with the remainder of the SGA group.

In one study[43] perinatal cerebral distress was used to define high-risk status. The definition of perinatal cerebral distress was not specified in the report, although it was stated that the most frequently listed diagnoses in these children were hyaline membrane disease, 1–minute Apgar score ≤3, apnea, and bradycardia. Also mentioned as occurring with some frequency were perinatal depression or asphyxia, pneumothorax, atelectasis or lung collapse, persistent fetal circulation, persistent ductus arteriosus, and cardiac arrest. Outcomes were neurologic functioning at 3 and 6 months of age and Bayley developmental scores at 12 months. Sample sizes were small, particularly at 12 months. Statistical tests were not performed for the 12–month outcomes. A preterm SGA high-risk group and a mixed full-term/preterm (proportion of each not reported) SGA low-risk group were included, as were a preterm AGA high-risk group, a preterm AGA low-risk group, and a full-term AGA low-risk control group. High-risk status as defined by perinatal cerebral distress appeared to be associated with poorer developmental outcomes for both the SGA and AGA preterm infants. Any high-risk versus low-risk comparison among the SGA infants in this study would be in part confounded by preterm or full-term status (i.e., for SGA infants, high-risk was represented only in preterm infants and low-risk only in the full-term/preterm group).

In a 10–year follow-up of infants with IUGR (birth weight at or below the 10th percentile for gestational age), a neonatal problems index was used in multiple regression analyses of potential predictors of intelligence test performance.[9] The neonatal problems index was the sum of the following: mechanical ventilation, exchange transfusion (regardless of number), respiratory distress syndrome, convulsions, apneic attacks (any number), systolic blood pressure below 40 mm Hg, evidence of fetal distress, edema (excluding orbital edema), 10% glucose therapy, 25% glucose therapy, bicarbonate therapy, Apgar score at 1 minute ≤3, and Apgar score at 5 minutes ≤5. This IUGR group included both preterm and full-term infants. The neonatal problems index did not differentiate intelligence test performance (verbal, performance, or overall IQ) within the IUGR sample. The number of neonatal problems was relevant, however, when children with IUGR were compared with control children whose birth weights were more than 2,500 gm and who were matched with the IUGR group for sex, ordinal position in the family, maternal smoking, maternal height, and social class. The intelligence test performance of the child with IUGR was found to be less impaired relative to that of the control subject if there was less difference in the number of neonatal problems between the children.

IMPORTANCE OF ASSOCIATED MEDICAL CONDITIONS AND THE POSTNATAL ENVIRONMENT

Associated Medical Conditions

Relatively little is known about how developmental outcome varies in infants with IUGR as a function of maternal and neonatal medical conditions experienced. Somewhat more information is available about associations between maternal and infant medical conditions and later development for other population groups.[2, 46–48]

Given the uncertainty of how various medical conditions relate to development in the IUGR population and the possibility that the infant with IUGR may be particularly vulnerable to some conditions,[49] it is important to consider both maternal and infant medical conditions in terms of developmental prognosis and follow-up care. Allen[2] has provided detailed recommendations regarding procedures for generating developmental prognoses for the infant with IUGR and for planning clinical follow-up of developmental progress.

Postnatal Environment of the Infant and Child

Environmental factors are known to relate both to the occurrence of IUGR and to a child's developmental performance (see Fig 4–1). Several studies have attempted some degree of accounting for environmental factors when examining relationships between IUGR and later development. Often this effort has entailed some type of matching of comparison groups using an indicator of socioeconomic status (e.g., parental occupation, parental education). These studies have an important methodologic advantage over those that took no account of environmental factors, but it must be recognized that socioeconomic status does not provide precise indication of the specific environmental experience of a child.[50, 51] Put another way, within a given socioeconomic level of the population, children certainly are exposed to variation in environmental experiences. A growing research literature documents relationships between aspects of the home environment (e.g., emotional and verbal responsivity of mother, avoidance and restriction of punishment, organization of the physical and temporal environment, provision of appropriate play materials, maternal involvement with the child, and opportunities for variety in daily stimulation) and children's cognitive development.[52] In addition there exists a body of research on parent-infant interactions, some of which suggests that at-risk infants may present different behavior patterns to parents and may have different social experiences with parents than do infants not at risk.[53–55]

It is quite possible that the relationships between newborn IUGR status and later development are influenced to a considerable degree by the post-natal experiences provided by the parents in the home environment and experiences provided by health and education services. For understandable practical reasons, studies of the later development of infants with IUGR have provided very little detailed information on the experiences of the children between birth and the ages at which the follow-up assessments were carried out.

In their follow-up of infants with IUGR to 5, 6, and 7 years of age, Neligan et al.[17] studied several variables that they labeled family factors, including measures of social class (father's occupation) and mother's care of the child (based on a home health visitor report when the child was 3 years old). The mothers' care of the child was rated as good, average, or poor based on adequacy of food, clothing, and supervision, the latter including the seeking of appropriate help in the case of illness and evidence of affectionate parental interest in the child. Although this measure of mother's care of the child was made up of diverse components, it nonetheless represented an attempt to assess environmental factors during follow-up. Also measured were biologic factors of mother and child and clinical factors of mother (antepartum hemorrhage, mode of delivery) and of child (delay in establishing regular respiration). From their multivariate analyses done separately for the VLFD group (birth weight below the 5th percentile for gestational age), the authors concluded that family factors accounted for the largest proportion of the variation in performance on development outcomes in this group of children with IUGR. These findings clearly indicate the importance of environment on later development in the child with IUGR. The considerable importance of environmental experiences was strongly suggested by Illsley and Mitchell[9] in their report on the childhood development of low birth weight infants and by Vohr and Oh[21] in the discussion of their findings regarding developmental performance in preterm SGA and preterm AGA children at 5 years of age.

Growth retarded infants and children are likely to experience variation in environmental experiences provided by parents, which in turn could influence the relationship between newborn IUGR status and later developmental status. In addition, a proportion of IUGR infants and children are likely to be involved in early intervention programs aimed at enhancing development by way of services to infants, young children, and parents.[56–58] If these programs are effective, they too could influence relationships between newborn IUGR status and later development.

SUMMARY

The realities of follow-up investigations necessitate caution in predicting later development in infants with IUGR. On the basis of available information, it appears that full-term infants with IUGR as a population group are not at high risk for major developmental deficits but may be at some risk for minimal cerebral dysfunction, including increased incidence of speech and language problems, minor neurologic findings, attention deficits, and school difficulties despite normal intelligence. Less is known about the development of preterm infants with IUGR. Limited attention has been given to possible explanatory mechanisms underlying relationships between IUGR and developmental outcomes. When this issue has been addressed explicitly, with some exceptions[59] the mechanisms discussed usually have been rather general (e.g., impaired brain growth, impaired fetoplacental function).

Subdividing the heterogeneous IUGR population into more homogeneous groups offers the potential to establish a better understanding of the development of these infants and therefore more accurate prognoses and more appropriate plans for postnatal services. Some attempts have been made to investigate the development of IUGR subgroups. Subgroups designated on the basis of timing of intrauterine insult have shown consistent findings across investigations, whereas findings for subgroups designated on the basis of maternal conditions during pregnancy and on the basis of neonatal medical conditions have shown some inconsistencies. The inconsistencies may in part be related to methodologic variations across investigations. There is need for continued efforts to examine IUGR subgroups, including attempts at basic differentiation of those infants whose IUGR status reflects normal adaptation to pregnancy conditions from those whose IUGR reflects pathologic insult.[60, 61] In predicting later development in an infant with IUGR, it is important to consider the infant's medical condition and the nature of the environment likely to be experienced during infancy and childhood.

ACKNOWLEDGMENTS

I thank Fay Menacker, R.N., P.N.P., for assistance in locating and evaluating materials for the preparation of this chapter, and Donald Cornely, M.D., David Heppel, M.D., and Jose Villar, M.D., for their critical reviews of drafts of the chapter.

REFERENCES

1. Kiely JL, Paneth N: Follow-up studies of low-birthweight infants: Suggestions for design, analysis and reporting. *Dev Med Child Neurol* 1981; 23:96.

2. Allen MC: Developmental outcome and followup of the small for gestational age infant. *Semin Perinatol* 1984; 8:123.
3. Susser M, Hauser WA, Kiely JL, et al: Quantitative estimates of prenatal and perinatal risk factors for perinatal mortality, cerebral palsy, mental retardation and epilepsy, in Freeman JM (ed): *Prenatal and Perinatal Factors Associated with Brain Disorders*. Bethesda, Md, National Institutes of Health, Publication No 85–1149, 1985, pp 359–439.
4. Low JA, Galbraith RS, Muir D, et al: Intrauterine growth retardation: A study of long-term morbidity. *Am J Obstet Gynecol* 1982; 142:670.
5. Kopp CB, McCall RB: Predicting later mental performance for normal, at-risk, and handicapped infants, in Baltes PB, Brim OG Jr (eds): *Life-Span Development and Behavior,* vol 4. Orlando, Academic Press, 1982, pp 33–61.
6. Ross G, Lipper EG, Auld AM: Consistency and change in the development of premature infants weighing less than 1,501 grams at birth. *Pediatrics* 1985; 76:885.
7. Fitzsimons RB, Ashby SA, Fitzhardinge PM: The prediction of school age I.Q. during infancy in the premature child. *Pediatr Res* 1978; 12:370.
8. Caputo DV, Mandell W: Consequences of low birthweight. *Dev Psychol* 1970; 3:363.
9. Illsley R, Mitchell RG: *Low Birth Weight: A Medical, Psychological and Social Study*. New York, John Wiley & Sons, 1984.
10. Rantakallio P, von Wendt L: Prognosis for low-birthweight infants up to the age of 14: A population study. *Dev Med Child Neurol* 1985; 27:655.
11. Starfield B, Shapiro S, McCormick M, et al: Mortality and morbidity in infants with intrauterine growth retardation. *J Pediatr* 1982; 101:978.
12. Koops BL: Neurologic sequelae in infants with intrauterine growth retardation. *J Reprod Med* 1978; 21:343.
13. Winer EK, Tejani NA, Alturu VL, et al: Four- to seven-year evaluation in two groups of small-for-gestational age infants. *Am J Obstet Gynecol* 1982; 143:425.
14. Villar J, Smeriglio V, Martorell R, et al: Heterogeneous growth and mental development of intrauterine growth-retarded infants during the first 3 years of life. *Pediatrics* 1984; 74:783.
15. Ounsted MK, Moar VA, Scott A: Small-for-dates babies at the age of four years: Health, handicap and developmental status. *Early Hum Dev* 1983; 8:243.
16. Chiswick ML: Intrauterine growth retardation. *Br Med J* 1985; 291:845.
17. Neligan GA, Kolvin I, Scott DMcL: Born too soon or born too small: A follow-up study to seven years of age. *Clinics in Developmental Medicine*, No 61. Philadelphia, JB Lippincott Co, 1976.
18. Commey JOO, Fitzhardinge PM: Handicap in the preterm small-for-gestational age infant. *J Pediatr* 1979; 94:779.
19. Fitzhardinge PM, Kalman E, Ashby S, et al: Present status of the infant of very low birth weight treated in a referral neonatal intensive care unit in 1974, in Ciba Foundation Symposium 59 (New Series): *Major Mental Handicap: Methods and Costs of Prevention*. New York, Elsevier North Holland, 1978, pp 139–150.
20. Vohr BR, Oh W, Rosenfield AG, et al: The preterm small-for-gestational age infant: A two-year follow-up study. *Am J Obstet Gynecol* 1979; 133:425.

21. Vohr BR, Oh W: Growth and development in preterm infants small for gestational age. *J Pediatr* 1983; 103:941.
22. Lipper E, Lee K, Gartner LM, et al: Determinants of neurobehavioral outcome in low-birth-weight infants. *Pediatrics* 1981; 67:502.
23. Hack M, Fanaroff AA, Merkatz IR: The low-birth-weight infant—evolution of a changing outlook. *N Engl J Med* 1979; 301:1162.
24. Fancourt R, Campbell S, Harvey D, et al: Follow-up study of small-for-dates babies. *Br Med J* 1976; 1:1435.
25. Harvey DR, Prince J, Bunton WJ, et al: Abilities of children who were small for dates at birth and whose growth in utero was measured by ultrasonic cephalometry. *Pediatr Res* 1976; 10:891.
26. Parkinson CE, Wallis S, Harvey D: School achievement and behaviour of children who were small-for-dates at birth. *Dev Med Child Neurol* 1981; 23:41.
27. Harvey D, Prince J, Bunton J, et al: Abilities of children who were small-for-gestational-age babies. *Pediatrics* 1982; 69:296.
28. Walther FJ, Ramaekers LHJ: Developmental aspects of subacute fetal distress: Behaviour problems and neurological dysfunction. *Early Hum Dev* 1982; 6:1.
29. Tanner JM, Thomson AM: Standards for birthweight at gestational periods from 32 to 42 weeks, allowing for maternal height and weight. *Arch Dis Child* 1970; 45:566.
30. Campbell S: An improved method of fetal cephalometry by ultrasound. *J Obstet Gynaecol Br Commonw* 1968; 75:568.
31. Campbell S, Newman GB: Growth of the fetal biparietal diameter during normal pregnancy. *J Obstet Gynaecol Br Commonw* 1971; 78:513.
32. Gross TL, Sokol RJ, Wilson MV, et al: Using ultrasound and amniotic fluid determinations to diagnose intrauterine growth retardation before birth: A clinical model. *Am J Obstet Gynecol* 1982; 143:265.
33. Kazzi GM, Gross TL, Sokol RJ, et al: Detection of intrauterine growth retardation: A new use for sonographic placental grading. *Am J Obstet Gynecol* 1983; 145:733.
34. Miller HC: Prenatal factors affecting intrauterine growth retardation. *Clin Perinatol* 1985; 12:307.
35. Villar J, Belizan JM: The timing factor in the pathophysiology of the intrauterine growth retardation syndrome. *Obstet Gynecol Surv* 1982; 37:499.
36. Hoffman H, Stark C, Lundin F, et al: Analysis of birth weight, gestational age and fetal viability, US births, 1968; *Obstet Gynecol Surv* 1974; 29:651.
37. Lubchenco LO, Hansman C, Boyd E: Intrauterine growth in length and head circumference as estimated from live births at gestational ages from 26 to 42 weeks. *Pediatrics* 1966; 37:403.
38. Low JA, Galbraith RS, Muir D, et al: Intrauterine growth retardation: A preliminary report of long-term morbidity. *Am J Obstet Gynecol* 1978; 130:534.
39. Leijon I, Billstrom G, Lind I: An 18–month follow-up study of growth-retarded neonates: Relation to neurobehavioural condition in the newborn period. *Early Hum Dev* 1980; 4:271.
40. Butler NR, Alberman ED (eds): *Perinatal Problems.* Edinburgh, E & S Livingstone, Ltd., 1969.
41. Ounsted M, Moar V, Scott WA: Perinatal morbidity and mortality in small-for-dates babies: The relative importance of some maternal factors. *Early Hum Dev* 1981; 5:367.

42. Westwood M, Kramer MS, Munz D, et al: Growth and development of full-term nonasphyxiated small-for-gestational age newborns: Follow-up through adolescence. *Pediatrics* 1983; 71:376.
43. Stave U, Ruvalo C: Neurological development in very-low-birthweight infants: Application of a standardized examination and Prechtl's optimality concept in routine evaluations. *Early Hum Dev* 1980; 4:229.
44. Usher R, McLean F: Intrauterine growth of live-born Caucasian infants at sea level: Standards obtained from measurements in 7 dimensions of infants born between 25 and 44 weeks of gestation. *J Pediatr* 1969; 74:901.
45. Ounsted M, Scott A, Moar V: Proportionality and gender in small-for-dates and large-for-dates babies. *Early Hum Dev* 1981; 5:289.
46. Wade RW, Searby J, Pepperell RJ, et al: Paediatric follow-up of pregnancies complicated by subnormal oestriol excretion. *Br J Obstet Gynaecol* 1985; 92:662.
47. Skouteli HN, Dubowitz LMS, Levene MI, et al: Predictors for survival and normal neurodevelopmental outcome of infants weighing less than 1001 grams at birth. *Dev Med Child Neurol* 1985; 27:589.
48. Low JA, Galbraith RS, Muir DW, et al: The contribution of fetal-newborn complications to motor and cognitive deficits. *Dev Med Child Neurol* 1985; 27:578.
49. Kyllerman M: Dyskinetic cerebral palsy. *Acta Paediatr Scand* 1982; 71:551.
50. Bradley RH, Caldwell BM: 174 children: A study of the relationship between home environment and cognitive development during the first 5 years, in Gottfried AW (ed): *Home Environment and Early Cognitive Development: Longitudinal Research*. Orlando, Academic Press, 1984, pp 5–56.
51. Wade RW, Pepperell RJ, Kitchen WH, et al: Paediatric follow up of pregnancies complicated by subnormal oestriol excretion: Interim report. *Med J Aust* 1978; 1:525.
52. Gottfried AW (ed): *Home Environment and Early Cognitive Development: Longitudinal Research*. Orlando, Academic Press, 1984.
53. Field TM: Interactions of preterm and term infants with their lower- and middle-class teenage and adult mothers, in Field TM, Goldberg S, Stern D, et al (eds): *High-Risk Infants and Children: Adult and Peer Interactions*. Orlando, Academic Press, 1980, pp 113–132.
54. Goldberg S, Brachfield S, DiVitto B: Feeding, fussing, and play: Parent-infant interaction in the first year as a function of prematurity and perinatal medical problems, in Field TM, Goldberg S, Stern D, et al (eds): *High-Risk Infants and Children: Adult and Peer Interactions*. Orlando, Academic Press, 1980, pp 133–153.
55. Kogan KL: Interaction systems between preschool handicapped or developmentally delayed children and their parents, in Field TM, Goldberg S, Stern D, et al (eds): *High-Risk Infants and Children: Adult and Peer Interactions*. Orlando, Academic Press, 1980, pp 227–247.
56. Bricker DD (ed): *Intervention With At-Risk and Handicapped Infants: From Research to Application*. Baltimore, University Park Press, 1982.
57. Frank M (ed): *Infant Intervention Programs: Truths and Untruths*. New York, The Haworth Press, 1985.
58. Simeonsson RJ, Cooper DH, Scheiner AP: A review and analysis of the effectiveness of early intervention programs. *Pediatrics* 1982; 69:635.

59. Brandt I: Brain growth, fetal malnutrition, and clinical consequences. *J Perinat Med* 1981; 9:3.
60. Read MS, Catz C, Grave G, et al: Introduction: Intrauterine growth retardation—Identification of research needs and goals. *Semin Perinatol* 1984; 8:2.
61. Warshaw JB: Intrauterine growth retardation: Adaptation or pathology? *Pediatrics* 1985; 76:998.

PART III

Etiology and Mechanisms

5

Maternal and Placental Causes of Intrauterine Growth Retardation

Thomas L. Gross, M.D.

When fetal growth retardation is suspected, a cause can be identified in only a minority of cases. Even after birth a cause for growth retardation in the small for gestational age neonate can be found in fewer than 50% of cases. Optimal management of any medical problem can only be achieved if the underlying cause can be diagnosed. In this chapter we examine maternal and placental causes of fetal growth retardation. However, prior to understanding abnormal fetal growth, some background information on normal fetal growth and development is necessary.

NORMAL FETAL GROWTH

Fetal Growth Curve

Figure 5–1 contrasts the average curves of fetal and placental growth and the change in amniotic fluid volume. In late gestation growth in the fetus slows, placental growth nearly stops, and the volume of amniotic fluid decreases. During the first half of pregnancy there is good agreement that the average fetal weight is about 5 gm at 10 weeks and 300 gm at 20 weeks. One of the most interesting aspects of the normal fetal growth curve is the appearance of a decline in fetal growth late in pregnancy. The most likely explanation for this is that there may be a normal decline in the supply of nutrients shunted transplacentally in late pregnancy, resulting in an expected slowing of growth. This is supported by the fact that the curve for the average

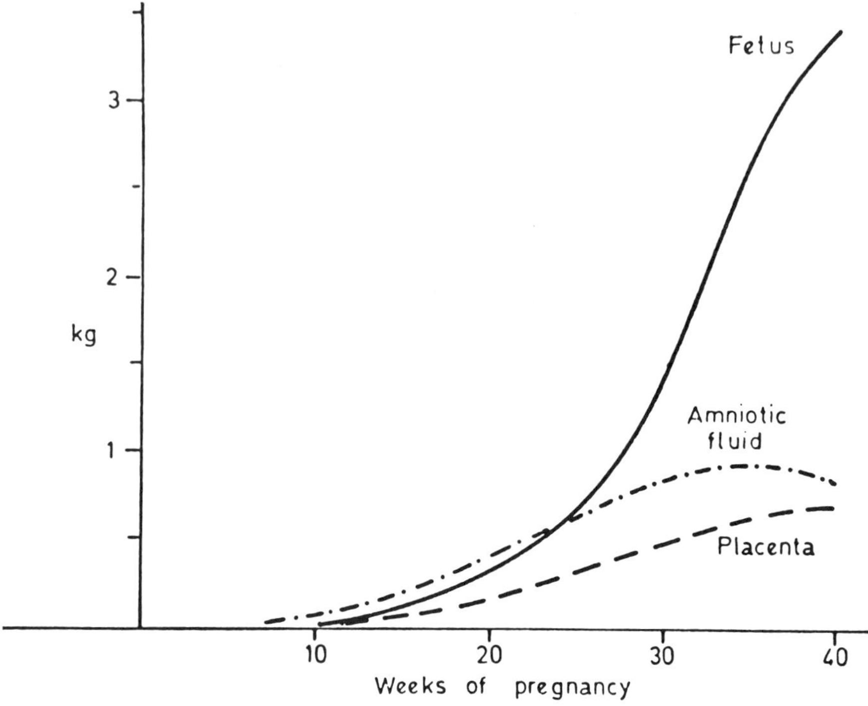

FIG 5–1.
Variation in fetal growth, amniotic fluid volume, and placental size with increasing gestation. (From Hytten FE, Leitch I: *The Physiology of Human Pregnancy.* London, Blackwell Scientific Publications, 1971. Used by permission.)

placental weight also plateaus late in pregnancy. However, this likely occurs only in certain at-risk pregnancies. In most patients fetal growth persists beyond term, and postdatism is commonly associated with macrosomia.

Substrates Used for Fuel for Fetal Growth

The substrates used by the fetus to supply energy for all of its functions, including growth, are shown in Table 5–1 for the sheep fetus, one of the few animal models studied thoroughly. There are indications that the percent of energy supplied by glucose may be even higher in the human fetus. Amino acids and ketone bodies cross the human placenta, and enzyme systems exist in the fetus that can use these substrates for energy. Selected free fatty acids also cross the human placenta, although transfer is slow (Fig 5–2). The overall contribution to fetal energy supply of the alternate fuels is probably not significant. Glucose serves as the major supplier for fetal growth, and because of this insulin is usually referred to as the fetal growth hormone.

TABLE 5–1.
Substrates Used for Fuel in the Fetus*

Substrate	Percentage of Total Fetal Energy Supply
Glucose	50
Amino acids	25
Lactate	20
Acetate	5
Free fatty acids	Not significant
Keto acids	Not significant

*Adapted from Milley JR, Simmons A: *Clin Perinatal* 1979; 6:365.

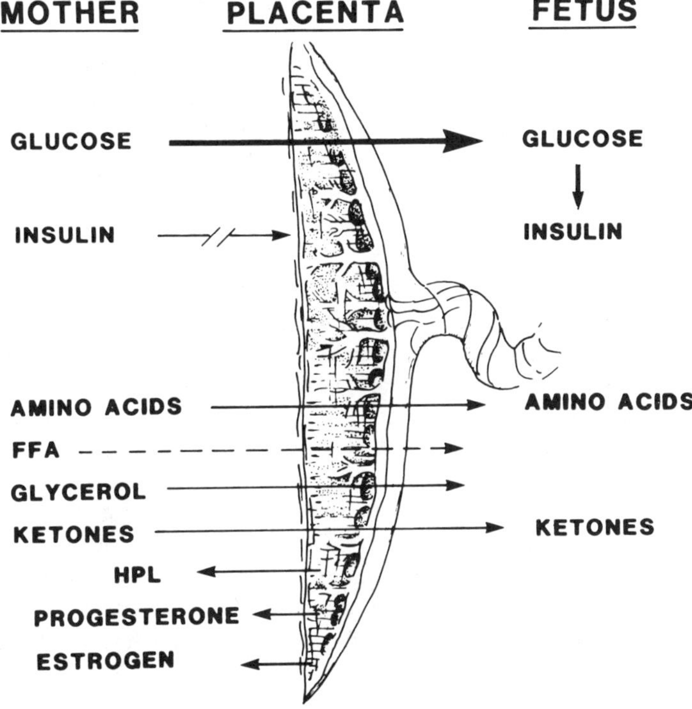

FIG 5–2.
Maternofetal transfer of fuels and placental production of hormones. Glucose, amino acids, glycerol, and ketones are transferred from mother to fetus. Free fatty acids are transferred to a limited extent. Insulin is not transferred, and insulin present in the fetus is produced by the fetal pancreas. Placental hormones, including human placental lactogen, estrogen, and progesterone, have known effects on maternal carbohydrate metabolism. (From Gross TL, in Gleicher N, Roux J (eds): *Principles of Medical Therapy in Pregnancy.* New York, Plenum Publishing Corp, 1985, pp 320–332. Used by permission.)

MATERNAL CAUSES OF FETAL GROWTH RETARDATION

Maternal Malnutrition

Normal Maternal Nutrition.—An additional 75,000 kcal is estimated to be required during a normal pregnancy. This includes the energy estimated to be needed for the additional maternal tissues added during pregnancy and for the tissue deposited in the fetus. The 75,000 kcal figure is calculated by simply estimating the amount of fat and protein laid down in maternal and fetal tissues and then converting it to energy. Of the 75,000 kcal, nearly 50% is accumulated as fat stores in the mother and fetus. If the increased need for calories were evenly divided over a 280-day gestation (which it is not), this would amount to an increased need of 270 kcal/day. This is rounded off to 300 kcal/day, the usual clinical recommendation for increased caloric need during a normal pregnancy.[1]

The estimate for increased protein needs during pregnancy is even more suspect. The increase varies between countries, from 5 gm/day in some European countries to 30 gm/day in the United States. There is really no clinically applicable research that can be applied to help determine the appropriate amount. Most nutritionists calculate that the pregnant woman needs 1.3 gm protein in her diet per kilogram lean body weight during pregnancy.

Maternal Weight Gain.—Virtually all major studies have found a strong positive association between both increasing prepregnancy maternal weight and maternal weight gain during pregnancy, and increasing birth weight in the offspring. Both increasing prepregnancy maternal weight and maternal gain during pregnancy are associated with higher mean birth weights and fewer low birth weight infants. Studies from the Collaborative Perinatal Project indicate that of the 30 maternal variables examined, prepregnancy weight and maternal pregnancy weight gain were the two strongest factors affecting birth weight.[2] Weight gain during pregnancy is usually more important as a determinant of birth weight than is maternal prepregnancy weight; however, the effect on birth weight of increasing maternal weight during pregnancy is strongest in smaller mothers, and is nearly lost in mothers weighing more than 190 pounds (Figs 5–3 and 5–4).

Energy Deprivation Versus Protein Deprivation.—Although it is well known that maternal malnutrition significantly increases fetal growth retardation, it is not clear whether the deprivation of maternal calories or of protein is more important.

Animal models can play a major role in differentiating the importance of energy and protein deficiency on fetal growth. However, it is not simple to separate the effects of carbohydrate and protein even in animals, because protein-deprived animals often eat less carbohydrate and thus confuse determination of which is causing the most severe growth retardation. Most

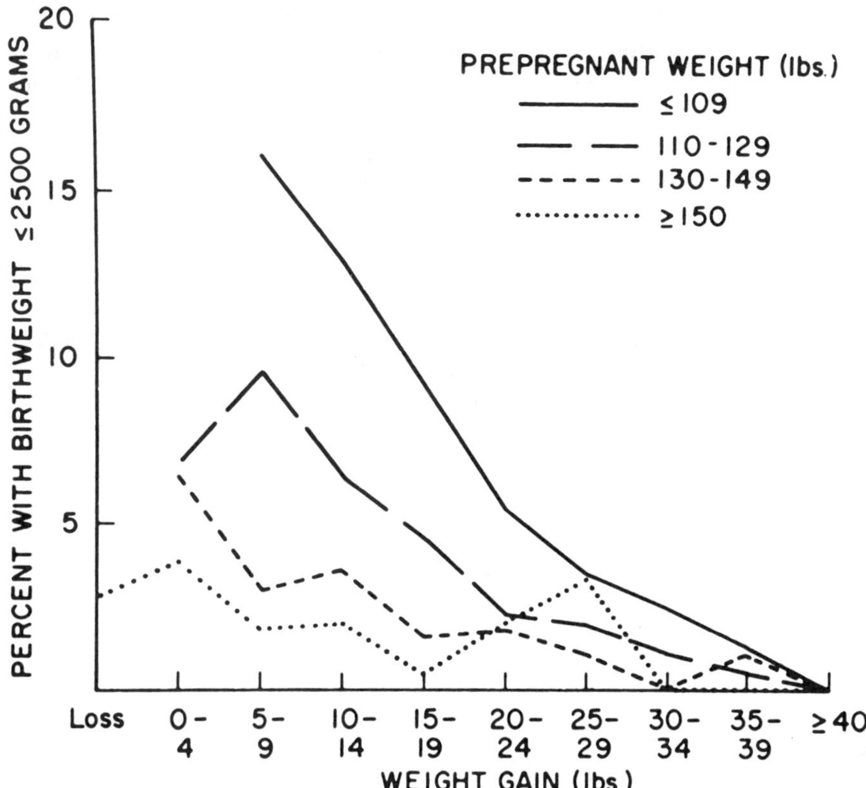

FIG 5–3.
Relationship of both prepregnancy maternal weight and maternal weight gain during pregnancy with the percent of low birth weight offspring. The major relationships between increased pregnancy weight gain and decreased low birth weight offspring is in underweight mothers. From Niswander KR, et al: *Obstet Gynecol* 1969; 33:482. Used by permission.)

investigators have concluded that it is the energy in the diet that plays the primary role in retarding fetal growth.

Human Studies of Hypoglycemia.—Hypoglycemia in the mother has been associated with fetal growth retardation and intrauterine death. However, this association with hypoglycemia has been poorly studied and must await confirmation in larger trials before applying it in the clinical setting.

Malnourished Mothers and Fetal Growth Retardation.—Several theories have been postulated as to why malnourished mothers may have more infants with fetal growth retardation. First, this may simply be related to less fuel being available for transplacental shunting to support fetal growth. Another recent suggestion is that the food-restricted mother may have decreased placental blood flow. Animal studies suggest that a 50% decrease in maternal diet can cause decreased blood volume in the mother, with a secondary decrease in cardiac output and a subsequent decrease in uterine blood flow. It is hypothesized that this declining blood volume with its effect on placental flow may be a major cause of fetal growth retardation in malnourished animals.

Teenage Mothers and Fetal Growth Retardation.—It has frequently been hypothesized that the teenage mother is at increased risk for delivering a growth-retarded infant, and in fact, teenage pregnancy is frequently cited as a risk factor for intrauterine growth retardation (IUGR). However, more recent information suggests that teenagers are not at increased risk for delivering infants with fetal growth retardation unless they have associated factors that are known to cause IUGR, such as poor prenatal care, poverty, poor nutrition, and use of illicit drugs, including alcohol and tobacco. When teen-

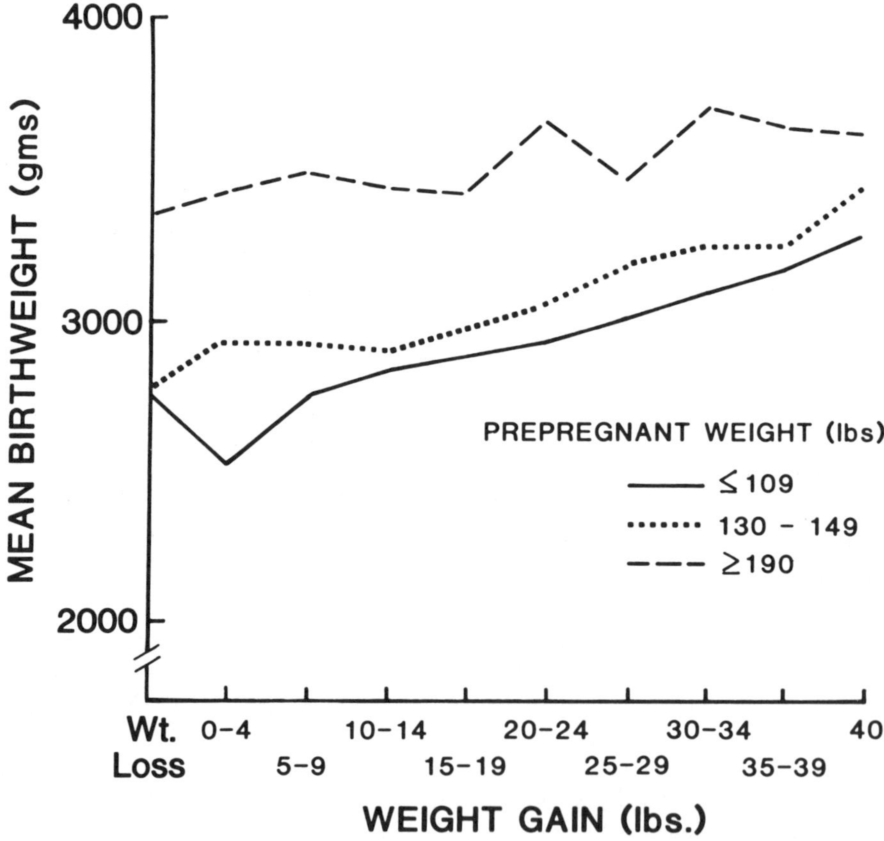

FIG 5–4.
Relationship of both prepregnancy maternal weight and maternal weight gain during pregnancy, and birth weight. The major effect of pregnancy weight gain and increasing birth weight is in women weighing less than 150 lb, and the effect is lost in obese mothers. (From Niswander KR, et al: *Obstet Gynecol* 1969; 33:482. Used by permission.)

agers are cared for in a setting of good prenatal care and counseling, teenage status alone does not increase the risk for fetal growth retardation.

Relationship of Poverty and Malnutrition.—Maternal malnutrition is usually associated with other factors that can have major effects on pregnancy outcome, such as maternal race, age, parity, height, general health, frequency of infections, education, genetic factors, and living and working conditions. A major confounding variable is poverty. Essentially, all patients who are chronically malnourished, except the occasional food faddist, are poor. In attempting to isolate the effect of maternal malnutrition on fetal growth and other complications, it is important to attempt to control for these confounding variables. At present it is impossible to isolate the effect of diet from the other variables.

Practical Maternal Nutritional Counseling.—There is no disagreement that severe maternal malnutrition can worsen pregnancy outcome, but the effects of less severe malnutrition are not so clear. Experts in nutrition will continue to search for the maternal diet associated with optimal pregnancy outcome, but for the present some practical guidelines[1] can be established that will allow clinicians to care for their patients in a fashion associated with excellent outcome.

1. Advise the healthy expectant mother to continue to eat a balanced diet. Food intake should be similar to that before pregnancy, with the addition of a quart of whole milk per day.
2. Question the patient to be certain food intake is adequate, particularly in patients of lower socioeconomic class.
3. Observe maternal weight gain during pregnancy to be certain the patient is gaining at a rate equivalent to approximately 25 lb for the entire pregnancy. Keep in mind that a wide range of weight gain is associated with normal outcome.
4. Question the patient throughout the pregnancy to uncover a history of food fads or other bizarre diets.
5. Women at highest risk for infants with growth retardation due to malnutrition are shown in Table 5–2. These patients should have a nutritional consultation at their first prenatal visit.
6. For underweight mothers the following guidelines are appropriate:
   a. Be more aggressive in obtaining a history of dietary intake and arranging formal dietary counseling.
   b. Give the patient formal dietary instructions including proper number of calories and amount of protein. It is imperative to prepare a dietary plan using foods the patient is familiar with. This is often forgotten even by nutritionists.

c. Provide nutritionally oriented follow-up sessions throughout the pregnancy.
d. There is no evidence that caloric intake beyond that recommended for normal mothers improves pregnancy outcome in underweight patients.

7. For overweight mothers the following guidelines are appropriate:
a. In mildly obese patients (greater than 120% but less than 150% standard weight for height), the usual weight gain and dietary intake for a normal pregnancy should be recommended.
b. In massively obese patients (greater than 150% standard weight for height), it can be definitely stated that the mother should not lose weight during pregnancy. The optimal amount of maternal weight gain during pregnancy is not clear, and some clinicians recommend the usual 24 to 28 pounds, but most physicians believe that 10 to 15 pounds is adequate.
c. Encourage the patient to lose excess weight postpartum.

Chronic Maternal Hypertension

Chronic maternal hypertension due to either essential hypertension or maternal renal disease can cause fetal growth retardation. The risk of fetal growth retardation increases as the maternal disease becomes more prolonged and severe, as manifested by high systolic and diastolic blood pressures, the duration of maternal disease, and the presence of vascular changes in other organs such as kidneys and eyes. The cause of IUGR in these patients is uncertain, but may represent a microvascular effect causing decreased uteroplacental blood flow. It may also be due to an abnormally small placenta, possibly related to a preexisting problem. The maternal vascular space increases by 50% in the normal pregnancy, but this has not been observed in many mothers with chronic hypertension. Such lack of increase in intravascular volume could cause a small placenta or decreased placental blood flow. It is also known that diuretics further decrease the intravascular volume, and this is the best reason not to use diuretics as therapy for chronic hypertension in the pregnant patient.

TABLE 5–2.
Women at High Risk for Infants With Growth Retardation Due to Malnutrition During Pregnancy

Women with low prepregnancy weight.
Women with inadequate weight gain during pregnancy.
Women with low income or for whom food purchase is an economic problem.
Women with a history of frequent pregnancies.
Women with a previous history of delivering infants with low birth weight.
Women with diseases known to cause nutritional problems, such as chronic infections, anemia, and drug addiction.
Women who are known to be vegetarians or have other abnormal diets.

The approach associated with the best outcome in the mother with chronic hypertension and her fetus is to use antihypertensive agents to control the maternal blood pressure near normal. Hydralazine (Apresoline) and methyldopa (Aldomet) are used most commonly, but for severe hypertension other agents are frequently needed, and beta blockers are now being used successfully.

Elevated blood pressure due solely to chronic hypertension is treated aggressively with antihypertensive agents. Hypertension secondary to toxemia and chronic hypertension plus toxemia are *not* treated with drugs. The blood pressure is controlled with bed rest if possible, and if the risk to the mother is too severe, the fetus is delivered.

Drugs of Abuse

Smoking.—In developed countries cigarette smoking is the most important known cause of fetal growth retardation. Smoking causes symmetric IUGR. On average, smoking decreases birth weight by 250 gm. The main effect of maternal smoking occurs in the third trimester. Thus women who stop smoking in the first or second trimester can be advised that smoking has not likely affected their infant's birth weight. Why smoking causes low birth weight is unknown, but the most likely mechanism is increased carboxyhemoglobin, resulting in decreased fetal oxygenation.

Alcohol.—IUGR is a major feature of fetal alcohol syndrome, with other findings including atypical facial appearance, developmental delay, and multiple anatomic defects. There is general agreement that heavy maternal alcohol intake places the fetus at risk for fetal alcohol syndrome, but the threshold amount of ethanol intake that can cause fetal effects is not known. Many studies show no effect of alcohol on fetal development in women drinking up to two drinks daily throughout pregnancy. When we determine the threshold at which alcohol is a risk, we may find that two drinks per day is the lower limit at which damage occurs, or we may eventually find that some women are more susceptible at even lower levels and that others can tolerate larger amounts of alcohol without development of fetal abnormalities.

When comparing the effects of alcohol and smoking, it is clear that maternal alcohol intake is not as consistent in retarding fetal growth as is maternal smoking.

Maternal Therapeutic Drugs

A very small group of therapeutic drugs is known to cause fetal growth retardation, among them phenytoin (Dilantin), sodium warfarin (Coumadin), and antimetabolites. Propranolol and other beta blockers have anecdotally been associated with fetal growth retardation, but have never been proved to be an actual cause.

Maternal TORCH Infections

TORCH (toxoplasmosis, rubella, cytomegalovirus, and herpes simplex) is a syndrome of nonbacterial infections that can cause severe fetal infection. All can cause severe fetal damage even when symptoms in the mother are minimal, and all can cause fetal growth retardation.

Maternal nonbacterial infections are commonly sought as a cause of fetal growth retardation. TORCH titers are frequently evaluated in high-risk patients; however, these infections are rarely proved as the cause of pregnancy complications. Cytomegalovirus infection is the most important.

Cytomegalovirus.—Maternal infection at any time in a pregnancy can result in hematogenous spread, with the virus invading the placenta, causing villitis, then gaining access to the fetus. Symmetric IUGR, deafness, mental retardation, and delayed psychomotor development can result if infection occurs before the third trimester. The retarded fetal growth may be the result of declining blood flow due to placentitis and cellular necrosis or may be related to a direct effect of the virus on fetal tissue. Mothers infected before pregnancy can also deliver infected neonates, although these infants are not as severely affected as those of mothers with first-trimester infection.

Diagnosis of cytomegalovirus as a cause of IUGR begins with demonstration of IgG and IgM antibodies in maternal blood. The presence of IgG antibodies means the mother has been infected at some time in her life; IgM antibodies signal a more recent infection. To make a definite diagnosis of maternal infection, the virus must be isolated from body secretions, and maternal urine and cervical cultures for cytomegalovirus are part of the workup when evaluating the mother for this infection. Definitive diagnosis of fetal infection can be made only by measuring the antibodies from umbilical cord blood or by culturing the virus from the amniotic fluid.

There is no proved therapy for cytomegalovirus infection diagnosed in mother and fetus.

For additional maternal and placental factors associated with IUGR, see Tables 5–3 and 5–4.

CONCLUSION

The recognition that not all low birth weight neonates are premature but that some are small because of inadequate growth in utero has been recognized for 25 years. However, a cause for fetal growth retardation can be identified in only a small group of mothers during pregnancy, and in only 50% of small neonates. The causes of IUGR must be sought intensely, because many of them require major management changes and also have implications for the infant's future development.

TABLE 5–3.
Maternal Conditions Associated With IUGR

Malnutrition
Medical problems
Chronic hypertension
Chronic renal disease
Collagen vascular disease
Hemoglobinopathies
SS Hemoglobin
Cyanotic heart disease
Thyrotoxicosis
Preeclampsia
Drugs of abuse
Tobacco
Alcohol
Heroin
Methadone
Phencyclidine (PCP)
Therapeutic drugs
Antimetabolites
Phenytoin
Steroids
Warfarin
Trimethadione
Infection
Cytomegalovirus
Rubella
Syphilis
Toxoplasmosis

TABLE 5–4.
Placental Disorders Associated With IUGR

Chorioangioma
Chronic abruptio placenta
Hydatidiform degeneration
Partial molar pregnancy
Single umbilical artery
Twin-to-twin transfusion syndrome

REFERENCES

1. Gross TL, Kazzi GM: The effects of maternal malnutrition and obesity on pregnancy outcome, in Gleicher N, Roux J (eds): *Principles of Medical Therapy in Pregnancy*. New York, Plenum Publishing Corp, 1985, pp 332–351.
2. Niswander KR, Singer J, Westphal M, Jr, et al: Weight gain during pregnancy and prepregnancy weight. *Obstet Gynecol* 1969; 33:482.

6

Intrinsic Causes of Fetal Growth Retardation: The Genetic Component

Mark I. Evans, M.D.

A 27-year-old gravida 2, para 1, white woman came for prenatal care at 12 weeks gestation. Her history and results of physical examination were normal, and uterine size was consistent with dates. Fetal growth was considered normal until 28 weeks, and a sonogram at 24 weeks had been consistent with dates. From 28 to 34 weeks fetal growth slowed; fundal height at 34 weeks was only 30 cm. Follow-up was with nonstress testing until 37 weeks, when fundal height was 32 cm. At that time a nonstress test was nonreactive and an oxytocin challenge test was positive. Cesarean section was performed. The 2100-gm female infant had rocker-bottom feet, low-set ears, and an abnormal thumb; apgar scores were 2 at 1 minute and 6 at 5 minutes. Karyotyping of the neonate's lymphocytes revealed a trisomy of chromosome 18. The baby died at 1 week of age.

Classically (and not appropriately), intrauterine growth retardation (IUGR) has been divided into two types.[1] Type I is referred to as symmetric growth retardation and is said to represent the result of intrinsic factors. Type II, or asymmetric growth retardation, is said to represent external factors, usually placental insufficiency, which most often leads to so-called brain-sparing IUGR. In Chapter 5 causes of IUGR that can be attributed specifically to external factors, such as maternal medical conditions or placental defects, are defined. In this chapter, as illustrated in the above case, we examine intrinsic conditions in the fetus, including genetic and infectious causes of fetal growth retardation.

It is well known that genetic disorders can lead to the development of a fetus with mild to severe IUGR. In general, the more "proportionate" the IUGR the earlier the onset, and therefore the higher the likelihood of a genetic cause. Whenever IUGR is suspected, the differential diagnosis of a fetal genetic disorder must also be considered; its presence, if confirmed, may alter clinical management. Such alterations in management may be indicated before, during, and also after delivery. It has been estimated that in perhaps as many as 10% of intrauterine growth–retarded fetuses congenital anomalies or an underlying genetic disorder is the cause.[2] Because placental insufficiency is unlikely in patients with high socioeconomic status, there is probably an inverse correlation between the presence of the so-called risk factors and likelihood that IUGR in any given patient is genetic.

CHROMOSOMAL DISORDERS

In several chromosomal disorders IUGR is a characteristic feature and is the main prenatal manifestation (Table 6–1). Each of these disorders can be diagnosed by amniocentesis or earlier in pregnancy by chorionic villus sampling. Even today, in most of these fetuses IUGR is not diagnosed until after delivery, often after emergency cesarean section performed because of fetal distress. Perhaps the single most important point of this chapter is that the obstetrician think "genetic etiology" as a possible cause of IUGR and perform proper third-trimester amniocentesis or chorionic villus sampling to predict IUGR when appropriate.

TABLE 6–1.
Chromosomal Disorders Associated With IUGR

Common cytogenetic disorders
Trisomy 18
Trisomy 21
Trisomy 13
Rare cytogenetic anomalies
Ring 1
Partial trisomy 1q
Trisomy 4p
4 p−
4 q−
5 p− (cri du chat)
5 q−
Ring 9
Ring 18
18 p−
18 q−
Ring 21
Trisomy 22

The mechanism of poor fetal growth with some chromosomal anomalies is not understood. Some authors have speculated slower cell cycles in aneuploid tissue cultures, but translation into clinical IUGR is not clear, especially as some abnormal fetuses show no evidence of poor fetal growth.

Trisomy 18

Trisomy 18 is a fetal chromosome abnormality of particular interest because both IUGR and polyhydramnios may be manifested early in the third trimester. This combination of findings makes third-trimester amniocentesis or chorionic villus sampling for prenatal diagnosis a definitive option, and one that has been clearly underutilized.

The frequency of trisomy 18 is said to be approximately 1 in 6,000 to 1 in 8,000 live births in the general population. As with all trisomies, the incidence of trisomy 18 appears to increase with advancing maternal age. Characteristic anomalies associated with the disorder are sufficiently significant that more than 50% of all liveborn infants with trisomy 18 will die in the first 2 months of life, and 90% within 1 year. In addition, trisomy 18 is clearly overrepresented among cases of postdate pregnancy, late fetal death, and stillbirth. Among the more important physical manifestations are low birth weight, prominent occiput, low-set ears, meningomyelocele, webbed neck, abnormal thumb, positioning of the index finger to overlap the third finger on flexion, and rocker-bottom foot. Several internal anomalies can occur, notably in the kidneys, intestines, and heart.

The natural history of trisomy 18 in the third trimester is one of progressive fetal deterioration. Beginning with IUGR and polyhydramnios, the obstetrician may also encounter abnormal nonstress test results, low biophysical profile scores, and monitoring abnormalities during labor. During labor, fetal distress is manifested by bradycardia. Such heart rate alterations are common and often lead to emergency cesarean section. Schneider et al.[3] have reported that more than 50% of babies with trisomy 18 are delivered by emergency cesarean section, albeit for a fruitless outcome. In the author's opinion, if trisomy 18 is diagnosed before labor, fetal monitoring and cesarean section because of fetal indications can be ethically avoided.

Trisomy 21

Trisomy 21, or more commonly Down's syndrome, can cause IUGR, although to a degree usually less severe than that seen with trisomy 18. Smith and McKeown[4] reported diminution of mean birth weight in infants with Down's syndrome to 2,894 gm compared with 3,321 gm in cytogenetically normal infants. However, the weight reduction is usually too small to be a clinically useful warning sign. Several other studies have confirmed slightly lower birth weight in infants with Down's syndrome, although such premature babies actually tended to be heavier than a comparable control group. Thus the growth retardation in Down's syndrome appears to be of later onset than in other cytogenetic disorders. Although less often a cause of IUGR than trisomy 18, trisomy 21 is clearly more common overall, occurring in approximately 1 in 800 births. The incidence is strongly tied to advanced maternal age. Classic findings include the so-called mongoloid facies (brachycephaly with flat occiput), upward slanting palpebral fissures, low-set ears, high-arched narrow palate, hypotonia, characteristic dermatoglyphic pattern of ulnar loops, distal displacement of the axial triradius, and transverse (simian) palmar crease. Clinically significant cardiac anomalies are seen in as many as 50% of infants with Down's syndrome. Many of these children will require surgery to ensure survival. It is not possible to predict the severity of individual organ anomalies before birth; obstetric counseling must rely on the reported statistical distribution of abnormal findings, and of necessity leaves much to be desired.

Trisomy 13

Trisomy 13, or Patau's syndrome, has an incidence of approximately 1 in 5,000 and is also correlated with maternal age. Birth weight is said to average about 2,400 gm for a 39-week gestation, and falls between that expected with trisomy 18 and trisomy 21. Clinical dysmorphologic features include a pattern of cleft lip, cleft palate, postaxial polydactyly, microcephaly, micrognathia, hypotelorism, low hairline, and microphthalmia. Cranial deformities such as cyclopia are occasionally seen, and urinary tract malformations are common. Cardiac defects including ventricular septal defects, patent ductus arteriosus, and coarctation of the aorta are common. Two thirds of these infants will die by 6 months, and about 90% within 1 year.

Turner's Syndrome

Turner's syndrome (karyotype 45,X) is a chromosome abnormality commonly associated with IUGR. The syndrome occurs in approximately 1 in 10,000 liveborn female infants, perhaps because the 45,X karyotype is the single most common abnormal karyotype seen in spontaneous abortions. It is estimated that more than 99% of all fetuses with Turner's syndrome are aborted spontaneously. Approximately one third of newborn babies with Turner's syndrome weigh less than 2,500 gm. It is interesting that those patients with the 45,X karyotype with only ovarian dysgenesis rather than the full compliment of features of Turner's syndrome (e.g., webbed neck, barrel chest) have birth weights approximately 100 gm heavier than those with classic Turner's syndrome, despite a gestational period averaging 1 week less.

Prenatally, the most common indication of Turner's syndrome is the sonar evaluation of a large mass (cystic hygroma) on the fetal neck (Fig 6–1), which

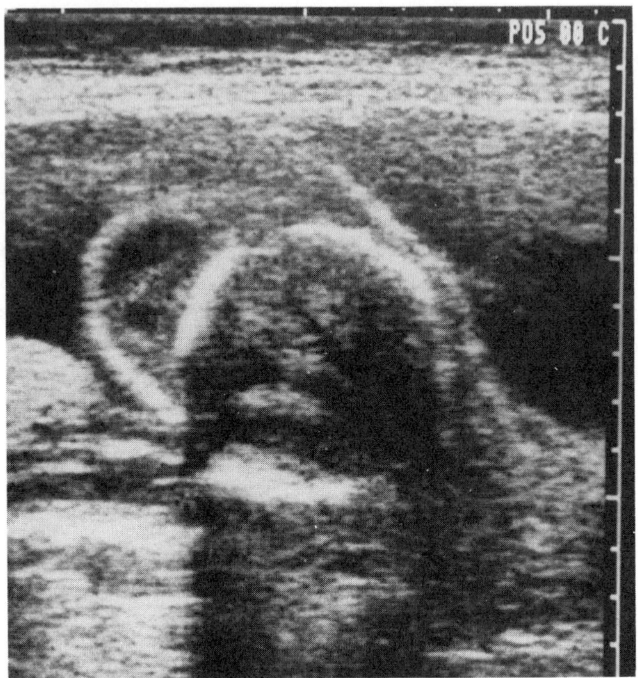

FIG 6–1.
Sonogram showing cystic hygroma on neck of fetus with Turner's syndrome.

partially obstructs the lymphatic drainage. Such a mass should be taken as indicating the presence of Turner's syndrome until proved otherwise. Cystic hygromas have occasionally been reported in association with trisomies.

The fetus with Turner's syndrome may have severe IUGR or be appropriate for gestational age. The most significant factors contributing to the variability in fetal weight of infants with Turner's syndrome are said to be the degree of mosaicism for other cell lines and other structural abnormalities of the X chromosome. Patients with mosaicism 45,X/46,XX tend to have higher birth weights than those with pure 45,X karyotype; however, those with an isochromosome of the long arm of X, e.g., 46Xi (Xq) often have lower birth weights than even those with pure 45,X. Furthermore, the probability of severe manifestations, including in utero fetal death or short stature, seems to be greater with pure 45,X than with a mosaicism. Short stature seems to be predominantly related to the absence of the short arm of the X chromosome (Xp); absence of the long arm (Xq) produces ovarian dysgenesis. In a liveborn female infant with Turner's syndrome, clinical phenomena may be sufficiently minimal (lymphedema, widely spaced nipples, webbed neck) to escape detection. In approximately 15% of liveborn infants a ventricular septal defect or coarctation of the aorta may also be found. If the diagnosis is not made before puberty is expected, the girl will usually come to the attention of a gynecologist because of primary amenorrhea and lack of secondary sexual characteristics.

If Turner's syndrome is diagnosed prenatally, the tremendous variability of phenotypic expression and range of IQ (most are normal) mandates extreme care in prenatal counseling. Frequently several meetings with counselors, physicians, and perhaps with affected children are necessary for thorough counseling. In general, prenatal diagnosis of Turner's syndrome is incidental to amniocentesis performed because maternal age is diagnosed because of abnormal α-fetoprotein or is secondary to ultrasound-defined growth anomalies, such as cystic hygroma. The management depends on the severity and findings. However, in the absence of growth anomalies, obstetric management must continue as for a fetus with a normal karyotype. A 45,X karyotype is not an indication for premature delivery or abortion of an otherwise viable third-trimester fetus. This philosophy does not preclude the mother from exercising her option of elective second-trimester termination prior to fetal viability.

Multiple Sex Chromosomes

Extra sex chromosomes (e.g., XXX found in 1 in 1,250 liveborn female infants and XYY found in 1 in 700 liveborn male infants) are more common than monosomies. Compilation of limited data on multiple sex chromosomes has suggested that birth weight decreases about 300 gm from the mean for each additional X chromosome. Although prenatal gravimetric influences of the extra sex chromosomes are open to interpretation, there are quantitative correlates to sex chromosome counts. There is an inverse correlation between fingertip ridge counts and sex chromosome number, with about 30 fewer for each X and 20 for each Y compared with control values. Rhodes et al.[5] have also inversely correlated intelligence (IQ) with the number of extra sex chromosomes, and suggest that an extra X correlates with −16 points and an extra Y with −5 points.

The clinical manifestations of extra sex chromosomes are usually more subtle than those of autosomal aneuploidy. As a result, prenatal counseling in those instances when second-trimester termination is feasible is extremely difficult. For the rare instance in which a third-trimester diagnosis might be made because of IUGR, complete obstetric care including intervention for fetal indications would seem warranted.

Miscellaneous Chromosomal Anomalies

In addition to the syndromes discussed, a variety of rare but reported cytogenetic anomalies can produce IUGR.[1] These conditions vary significantly in severity and in expected birth weight. Counseling and management must be individualized to the specific conditions and trimester when the diagnosis is made.

Low Maternal Serum α-Fetoprotein

Recent literature has clearly correlated low maternal serum α-fetoprotein levels and increased risk of aneuploidy. Such low levels may be a very safe marker by which to identify groups of patients not presently thought to be at high risk for aneuploidy who now may qualify for genetic amniocentesis. It has been estimated that perhaps as many as 40% of fetuses with Down's syndrome might be identified by low serum α-fetoprotein levels in women younger than age 35 years.[6] The use of maternal serum α-fetoprotein (MSAFP) has allowed maternal age counseling to be a function of both age and MSAFP value.[7] Cytogenetic abnormalities associated with low MSAFP occur in the same proportion as trisomies and other anomalies as seen in advanced maternal age.[8]

NEURAL TUBE DEFECTS

Neural tube defects are among the most common of the more serious congenital malformations. Failure of closure of the embryogenic neural tube results in anatomic anomalies ranging from a very small spina bifida to anencephaly. Neural tube defects are recognized as a group of disorders for which there are genetic and environmental causes. In the United States there are marked racial, geographic, and socioeconomic differences in incidence, with the highest occurrence among poor, white Appalachian patients.

Neural tube defects are divided into two major groups: anencephaly, that is, partial or complete absence of the cranium; and spina bifida with or without meningomyelocele, or failure of closure of the neural tube with possible extravasation of neural elements. The clinical findings vary, from uniform lethality in anencephaly to moderate to severe handicaps with spina bifida.

The diagnosis of neural tube defects is now often made prenatally. The anencephalic fetus is sometimes recognized as small for dates on fundal examination, prompting ultrasound examination. In addition, with the advent of commonplace, if not routine, use of ultrasonography, an increasing number of anencephalic fetuses are detected before birth.

Honnebier and Swaab[9] have documented lower growth rates for fetuses and placentas in anencephalic pregnancies, with growth decrements more obvious for birth weight than for placenta. Birth weight is usually less than the 25th birthweight percentile, although placental weight may be closer to the 50th percentile. Kolski et al.[10] reported a mean birth weight for anencephalic fetuses of 2,117 gm, compared with the norm of 3,204 gm in their Uruguayan population. There has also been a small number of twin pregnancies with one anencephalic and one normal fetus. Usually the anencephalic fetus has lower birth weight than the normal twin, even after adjusting for missing brain and bone weight.

Growth retardation in the spina bifida group is a less prominent clinical finding. Hydrocephalus is frequently present, causing a larger than expected fundal size and possible significant difficulties in delivery. Wald et al.[11] at Oxford found that male infants with spina bifida had a 200 gm weight decrement, and female infants a 240 gm decrement, compared with controls. Unlike trisomy 21, these decrements were not related to prematurity; fetuses with spina bifida were lighter than controls at all gestational ages.

The diagnosis of hydrocephalus can be made on ultrasound examination. The lesions of open spina bifida can be seen on detailed scanning; however, reliable visualization of small lesions requires highly trained personnel and advanced sonar equipment, and even an expert may fail to detect an open but flat lumbosacral defect.

It should be appreciated by obstetricians who perform their own in-office scans that difficulty in delineating the fetal skull during a routine scan may not be a technical artifact and that the diagnosis of anencephaly must be considered. Similarly, whenever a larger than expected head is seen, a detailed scan of the spine is in order.

Chemical screening for neural tube defects is now nearly universal in England and is becoming standard practice in the United States. In 1972 Brock and Sutcliffe[12] reported that when an open neural tube defect was present, levels of α-fetoprotein, a normal product of the fetal liver, were considerably elevated in amniotic fluid. Further work showed that maternal serum screening could define the population at high risk for neural tube defect and who thus required further investigation, including ultrasonography and amniocentesis.[13]

One by-product of maternal serum α-fetoprotein testing was an appreciation of the significance of elevated levels that eventually proved not to be related to neural tube defect or to other known causes, such as twin pregnancy, incorrect dates, or fetal death. From data collected by Wald et al.[11] and now others, in 25% of such cases the birth weight of the fetus was less than 2,500 gm. The cause of elevated maternal serum α-fetoprotein level with IUGR is unknown, but early placental dysfunction that may later manifest itself as IUGR is one hypothesis. In any event, as maternal serum α-fetoprotein screening for neural tube defect becomes more common in the United States, it may also become useful as a screening device for IUGR.

GENETIC DISORDERS OF BONE AND CONNECTIVE TISSUE

Several dwarfing disorders and deformities result in IUGR. Definitive prenatal diagnosis is possible for only some. For most, however, diagnosis is difficult even at birth, because frequently it is not until later in life that the diagnostic features of some diseases become manifest.

Dwarfing Syndromes

Achondroplasia is a common form of dwarfism in fetuses and adults. Genetic transmission may be either autosomal dominant or related to a spontaneous mutation often associated with advanced maternal or paternal age. Achondroplasia is not associated with severe fetal growth retardation; thus fetal achondroplasia is only occasionally diagnosed prenatally by late third-trimester ultrasonography or x-ray studies. The birth weight in sporadic cases is reported to be 3,300 gm. However, if the father has achondroplasia and the mother does not, birth weight of the affected fetus decreases by 300 gm. If the mother transmits the achondroplastic gene, birth weight is reduced by another 300 to 600 gm.[14] Cesarean section is usually the mode of delivery for a normal size infant from a mother with achondroplasia, because of cephalopelvic disproportion. The achondroplastic baby is often delivered by cesarean section to avoid damaging the spinal cord at the time of head extension at vaginal delivery.

In the instance of the homozygous "double dose" effect in a fetus who is the product of two parents with achondroplasia, severe IUGR is present and diagnosable either by x-ray or ultrasound studies. Such fetuses most often die either in utero or as neonates for reasons that are unclear.

Hypochondroplasia and cartilage hair hypoplasia are milder forms of achondroplasia. Data on birth weight are unreliable, and prenatal diagnosis is not yet possible.

Russell-Silver syndrome results in dwarfism in which there is subnormal growth velocity, clinodactyly (bent fingers), simian creases, triangular facies, genitourinary abnormalities, and type I IUGR. However, these children usually have normal intelligence. The genetics of the syndrome have not been delineated. At the very least, careful observation in subsequent pregnancies after the birth of an infant with Russell-Silver dwarfism would allow for presumptive prenatal diagnosis. Evans et al.[15] have recently diagnosed Langer-type mesomelic dwarfism by ultrasonography on the basis of disproportionate shortening of the distal compared with the proximal extremities beginning in the second trimester. With increasing sophistication of electronic hardware, such diagnosis should become more common.

The Chondrodystrophies

In contrast to the more common "achondroplasia-like" syndromes, which are usually compatible with life, are several disease entities that result in stillbirth or in death in the neonatal period or early infancy. Among these are achondrogenesis types I and II; the short rib, polydactyly syndromes such as Noonan-Saldino, Majewski, and Verma-Naumoff syndromes, with short ribs & polydactyly; thanatophoric dysplasia; and infantile forms of osteopetrosis, hypophosphatasia, and type II osteogenesis imperfecta.[1] In other chondrodystrophies, such as chondroectodermal dysplasia (Ellis–van Creveld syndrome) and asphyxiating thoracic dysplasia, the prognosis for neonatal survival is better. These syndromes may or may not be associated with IUGR, but rigorous ultrasonography may reveal thoracic compression, polydactyly, and short limbs. It should be noted, however, that although the fetus may be growth retarded, a large fundus secondary to polyhydramnios is often the diagnostic clue for further investigation.

Osteogenesis Imperfecta

Osteogenesis imperfecta is not a single disorder but more properly a class of genetic disorders characterized by molecular derangements of collagen leading to osteoporosis and greater than normal susceptibility to fractures. Genetic transmission is either autosomal dominant or recessive depending on the type. Of interest here is osteogenesis imperfecta type II, sometimes called lethal perinatal osteogenesis imperfecta syndrome, which is autosomal recessive and has a general population incidence of 1 in 60,000. These infants usually have IUGR; are born prematurely; and have short, broad thighs extending at right angles to the trunk and short, curved, deformed limbs. Birth weight for infants with osteogenesis imperfecta has been reported as averaging 1,500 gm at 37 weeks gestation. As with many of the chondrodystrophies, which are autosomal recessive disorders, prenatal diagnosis without prior history for a high index of suspicion is unlikely. However, in patients at high risk, diagnosis by x-ray evidence of fracture and short limbs is possible during the third trimester. If the diagnosis is made and the parents have been counseled regarding the fatal prognosis for the fetus, labor management may deliberately exclude performance of cesarean section because of fetal indications. There is little documentation of such practice, and the physician always risks community and potential legal ire when such a decision is made. The value of appropriate ethical and legal consultation cannot be overstressed.

Type III osteogenesis imperfecta, also autosomal recessive, is not as severe as type II, although occasionally intrauterine fractures are observed. The sclera are blue at birth, but become white if the child survives into adolescence. Intrauterine size and growth are probably within the normal range, but the same guidelines for management of high risk cases apply as with osteogenesis imperfecta type II.

Primordial Short Stature

Several other syndromes are manifested by IUGR. Their inheritance is uncertain, but is thought by some researchers to be autosomal recessive. These include Bloom's syndrome, in which there is hypoplasia of facial bones and telangiectasia of exposed areas, with the underlying defect being the cell's inability to repair DNA broken by ultraviolet irradiation from sunlight. Birth weight averages 1,972 gm and is among the lowest in genetic disorders compatible with survival.[16] Other rare disorders include the Seckel, Donohue, Cochayne, Cornelia de Lange, and Smith-Lemli-Opitz syndromes.

It is also likely that some inborn errors of metabolism, such as the sphingolipidoses, mucolipidoses, anemias (e.g., sickle cell and thalassemia), and immune deficiencies, often result in retarded growth. However, these conditions do not characteristically demonstrate a significant pattern of IUGR that would make any of them distinguishable by poor fetal growth.

THIRD TRIMESTER CYTOGENETIC DIAGNOSIS

The management of IUGR in the antepartum and intrapartum periods is described in later chapters. A few comments are appropriate here, however, with regard to the assessment of the genetic causes of IUGR. Patients with none of the well-known risk factors for asymmetric IUGR, such as maternal hypertension or malnutrition, are more likely to have a genetic defect.[1] Some authorities have estimated that perhaps 5% to 10% of cases of IUGR have an underlying genetic cause. This is increased when IUGR is seen in white patients of upper socioeconomic class, who are less likely to have maternal causes for fetal growth retardation.[2] Part of differential diagnosis between types I and II IUGR depends on the symmetry of the growth (Is there brain sparing or not?) and the timing of the insult.

Genetic amniocentesis is most commonly performed during the second trimester, but is also appropriately performed in the third trimester of pregnancy when there is strong clinical suspicion of a fetal chromosomal defect. Such procedures have classically been underutilized, partly because of the belief that chromosome karyotypes in the third trimester are difficult to obtain. Recent data have suggested that in fact there is not a substantial difference in the amount of time necessary to obtain the karyotype in the third trimester. With the advent of enriched culture media, the time required to achieve a diagnosis has been reduced substantially, and very often such data are available before clinical decisions must be made.[17] Similarly in those centers where chorionic villus sampling is performed, third trimester villi can be used for cytogenetic studies. In addition, fetal blood obtained by cordocentesis can be used for cytogenetic diagnosis. In experienced hands these are procedures with low morbidity. The results are available rapidly and so will likely be used more frequently in the future.[18]

There may be much controversy over the management of third-trimester fetuses shown to have IUGR secondary to an underlying genetic defect. Physicians in these difficult situations will be subjected to significant pressures, including moral, ethical, and legal questions. It is not clear at this writing what the standard of management in such cases will be over the next several years. However, despite the controversy that will no doubt be present, it is my position that the more knowledge that is obtained about a given clinical situation, the more intelligent the decision that can be made regarding management.

SUMMARY

1. It is very difficult to reliably diagnose IUGR in the antepartum period.
2. When IUGR is suspected either earlier than usual in gestation or in a patient who would not ordinarily be considered in a high-risk group based on maternal causes, the likelihood of a genetic defect is considerably increased.
3. Third-trimester cytogenetic diagnosis may be of tremendous utility in determining patient management, and should be considered in certain patients with severe IUGR.
4. Low maternal serum α-fetoprotein levels will identify a large cohort of patients who may be at higher than average risk for chromosomal anomalies. Elevated MSAFP not associated with a neural tube defect may reflect early placental dysfunction and an increased risk for subsequent fetal growth retardation.

REFERENCES

1. Lin CC, Evans MI: *Intrauterine Growth Retardation*. New York, McGraw-Hill Book Co, 1985.
2. Creasy R: Intrauterine growth retardation related to research and clinical application. Presented at the Tenth World Congress of Gynecology and Obstetrics, San Francisco, 1982.
3. Schneider AS, Mennuti MT, Zackai EJ: High cesarean section rate in trisomy 18 births: A potential indication for late prenatal diagnosis. *Am J Obstet Gynecol* 1981; 140:367.
4. Smith A, McKeown T: Prenatal growth of mongoloid defectives. *Arch Dis Child* 1955; 30:257.
5. Rhodes K, Markham RL, Maxwell PM, et al: Immunoglobulins and the X-chromosome. *Br Med J* 1969; 3:439.
6. Merkatz IR, Nitowsky HM, Macri JN, et al: An association between low maternal serum α-fetoprotein and fetal chromosomal abnormalities. *Am J Obstet Gynecol* 1984; 148:886.
7. Evans MI, Belsky RL, Greb A, et al: Maternal serum alpha-fetoprotein screening. *J Clin Assay* 1988; 10:210.
8. Drugan A, Dvorin E, Koppitch FC, et al: Counseling for low maternal serum alpha-fetoprotein should emphasize all chromosome anomalies, not just Down syndrome. *Obstet Gynecol* (in press).
9. Honnebier WJ, Swaab DF: The influence of anencephaly upon intrauterine growth of fetus and placenta and upon gestational length. *J Obstet Gynaecol* 1973; 80:577.
10. Kolski R, Mane-Garzon F, Seuanez H: Estudio de 56 casos de anencefalia en el Uruguay. *Arch Pediatr Uruguay* 1977; 48:209.

11. Wald N, Cuckle H, Stirret EM, et al: Maternal serum alpha-fetoprotein and low birth weight. *Lancet* 1977; 2:268.
12. Brock DJH, Sutcliffe RG: Alpha-fetoprotein in the antenatal diagnosis of anencephaly and spina bifida. *Lancet* 1972; 2:197.
13. Brock DJH, Bolton AE, Managhan JM: Prenatal diagnosis of anencephaly through maternal serum alpha-fetoprotein measurements. *Lancet* 1973; 2:923.
14. Murdoch JL, Walker VA, Hall JG, et al: Achondroplasia: A genetic and statistical survey. *Am J Hum Genet* 1970; 33:227.
15. Evans MI, Quigg MH, Zador IE, et al: Prenatal diagnosis and pathology of Langer type mesomelic dwarfism. *Am J Hum Genet* 1985; 37S:A225.
16. German J: Bloom's syndrome. I: Genetic and clinical observations in the first twenty patients. *Am J Hum Genet* 1970; 33:227.
17. Evans MI, Bhatia RK, Bottoms SF, et al: Effects of karyotype, gestational age, and medium on amniotic fluid cell culture duration. *J Reprod Med* (in press).
18. Evans MI, Schulman JD: Prenatal diagnosis: Invasive techniques and alpha-fetoprotein screening, in Avery GB (ed). *Neonatology: Pathophysiology and Management of the Newborn,* ed 3. Philadelphia, JB Lippincott, 1987, pp 130–138.

7

Intrauterine Growth Retardation in Twins

Richard A. Bronsteen, M.D.
Federico E. Mariona, M.D.
Robert J. Sokol, M.D.

Antenatal detection of a multiple gestation marks a pregnancy as a special event. Certainly for the parents the pregnancy seems to take on a special aura. For the physician there are extra concerns because of the higher incidence of complications for both fetus and mother. A frequent complication is intrauterine growth retardation (IUGR). As with singleton gestations, there are a variety of causes for suboptimal growth in twins; most are not specific for multiple gestation.

In this chapter we review growth retardation in twins by first describing the intrauterine growth normally seen in twin gestations. Then pathologic growth, its clinical significance, and diagnosis are discussed. The majority of papers in the literature on multiple gestations focus on twins. Though we will be limiting our discussion here to twin gestations, the principles are applicable to higher order multiple gestations (triplets, quadruplets, and above).

TWIN INTRAUTERINE GROWTH

Intrauterine growth has usually been studied through birth weight records, with preterm deliveries serving as standards for preterm intrauterine weights. Numerous reports in the literature are based on a wide variety of

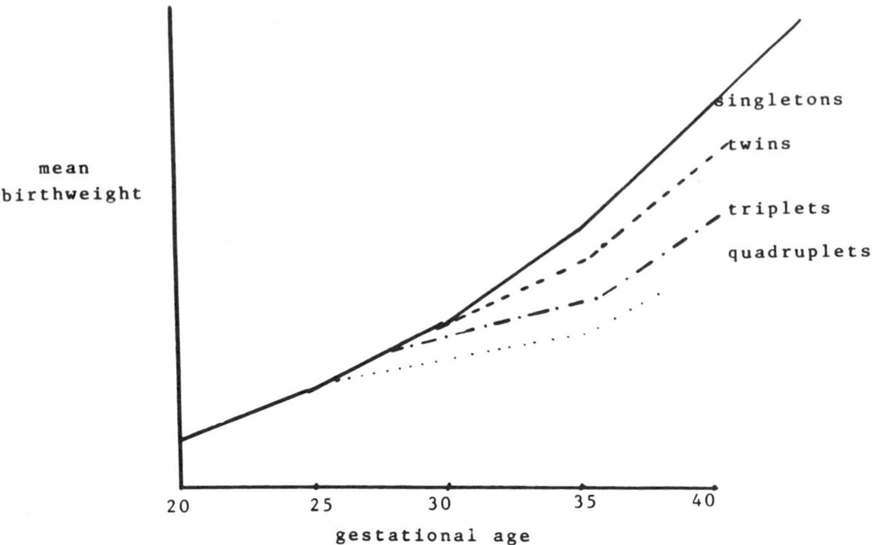

FIG 7–1.
Correlation of birth weight with gestational age. The higher the fetal number the lower the birth weight.

patient populations detailing the growth patterns in twins. The patterns are similar regardless of race or nationality studied; fetuses from multiple gestations are smaller than those of singleton gestations.

In an early study McKeown and Record[1] showed that as the number of fetuses increased, deviation from normal singleton growth also increased. As the number of fetuses increased from twins to triplets to quadruplets, the gestational age at which birth weight first fell below that of a singleton fetus decreased. Twins were found to have birth weights similar to singletons up to 30 weeks, and thereafter were below singleton levels. Similarly, birth weight in triplets fell off the singleton curve at 27 to 28 weeks, and in quadruplets at approximately 26 weeks. In addition, as the fetal number increased, the rate of individual fetal growth in the third trimester decreased. Thus the farther a multiple gestation advanced and the higher the fetal number, the greater the individual birth weight will differ from singleton values. These findings are shown schematically in Figure 7–1. Similar results have been obtained from other studies, with twin birth weights falling off the normal singleton curve at various times ranging from 30 weeks[2,3] to 32 weeks[4] to 33 weeks.[5]

Studies have also followed twin intrauterine growth with ultrasound scans. Unlike birth weight studies, these studies do not show a consistent pattern of growth. Studies evaluating biparietal diameter (BPD) have shown varied results, with BPD lagging behind singleton measurements in the mid–third trimester[4] to equivalent to singleton levels throughout gestation[6] and to smaller than singletons at all gestational ages.[7] We must use caution in drawing conclusions from these studies, however, because BPD is a poor predictor of weight in singletons, and its accuracy in twins is even worse.

Usually twins grow at nearly identical rates; the mean twin birth weight difference is 11%.[8] Fetuses small for gestational age (SGA) are found in 24% to 40% of twin gestations.[9–13] In one study, 13% of twin gestations resulted in one SGA fetus and 9.4% produced two SGA babies.[8]

ETIOLOGY OF DECREASED INTRAUTERINE GROWTH: PATHOLOGIC OR PHYSIOLOGIC?

It is widely accepted that twins are smaller than singletons of similiar gestational age. An appropriate question in the absence of any factor that could be responsible for the lower birth weight (such as a congenital or chromosomal anomaly) is whether this smaller size is pathologic (due to abnormal growth) or physiologic (due to smaller growth potential of twins). This is important in choosing an appropriate growth chart for either ultrasound measurements or birth weights with which to evaluate the twins.

As with singletons, the intrauterine growth of twin fetuses is determined by a combination of factors, both maternal and fetoplacental. Important determinants of intrauterine growth of singletons can also be expected to have an effect on twin intrauterine growth. In addition, several other factors specific to multiple gestation also play a role in determining birth weight.

Maternal Factors

The ability of the mother to supply the extra nutrients needed for two growing fetuses has a limiting effect on intrauterine growth. As with singletons, low parity, low maternal weight, and maternal smoking can all negatively influence fetal birth weight. These factors have all been found to exert their negative influence independent of the presence of twins.[14, 15] In addition, when comparing twins with singletons, maternal parity has a greater effect than does fetal sex on birth weight, suggesting a more crucial role of nutrient supply in twins.

Placental Factors

The type of placenta present in twins can also influence fetal growth. Birth weight studies have consistently shown that twins with dichorionic placentas are heavier than their monochorionic counterparts.[16, 17] Within the dichorionic group, unfused placentas yield babies with higher birth weight than do fused dichorionic placentas.[17] Abnormal umbilical cord insertions can adversely affect birth weight. With multiple gestations the incidence of velamentous and marginal insertions is increased, and these are associated with smaller infants. Decreases in placental blood flow and nutrient exchange from the different placental types and cord insertions are probably at least partially responsible for the lower birth weight.

Fetal Factors

Fetal factors also play a role in determining birth weight. Fetal sex influences birth weight, with male infants weighing more than female infants. Fetal zygosity influences birth weight, with monozygotic twins weighing less than dizygotic twins.[16, 17] Twins of different sex (all dizygotic with varied types of placentas) have been found to weigh more than same sex twins (mixed placental types and zygosity). The roles of fetal sex and zygosity can be difficult to distinguish, because the heavier groups in both instances contain only the more favorable dichorionic placentation. It is believed, though, that when gestational age, fetal sex, and placental type are controlled,[16] zygosity does influence fetal weight.

These studies illustrate pathologic reasons for lower twin birth weights. Are there data to also support a lower growth potential in twins? This is most pertinent for monozygotic twins, where splitting of the embryo may result in smaller fetuses due to the smaller cell number present in each of the resulting twin embryos. Data on monoamniotic monochorionic twins, where the late time of embryo splitting would be predicted to result in the smallest cell number in each of the embryos, show these neonates to be smaller than other twins at birth (2.1 kg mean birth weight versus 2.4 kg).[18] Data on these twins, though, are limited by the low frequency of monoamniotic twin births, and the smaller birth weights may also be the result of other pathologic causes.

Limited experimental studies on mouse embryos do not support the limited growth potential theory. Embryo cell number has no effect on birth weight. Experimental manipulation of early embryos such that their cell numbers are increased or decreased has no effect on eventual weight. The embryos undergo a growth regulation process, and normal weights for the species are found.[19, 20]

Anthropometric data suggest that the smaller twin weights are the result of asymmetric IUGR, because birth weight is the primary neonatal parameter that is decreased in twins. Although twin birth weight is lower than normal singleton values, both body length and head circumference are within normal singleton limits.[6] After delivery there is a period of rapid catch-up growth, and many growth-retarded fetuses reach normal size by infancy.[21]

In summarizing the studies on twin birth weight, the evidence suggests that the lower birth weights in twins are predominantly the result of pathologic processes. IUGR is a major reason for the smaller birth weights seen in twins. The evidence does not conclusively rule out the possibility that some of the decrease in birth weight is physiologic, resulting from smaller cell number, but this does not appear to be a major determinant of eventual twin birth weight. Even without the data, it is easy to understand why twins, with their increased nutrient demand on the maternal support system, would be more likely than singletons to be growth retarded.

OTHER PATHOLOGIC CAUSES OF IUGR IN TWINS

In addition to growth retardation resulting from a suboptimal nutrient supply, other factors can also play a role in determining twin birth weight, and many of these occur with increased frequency in multiple gestations.

Congenital malformations and genetic abnormalities can both occur in one or both twins. A recent review has summarized the findings of studies on congenital malformations in twins.[22] Although not all studies agree, it is believed that anomalies occur more frequently in twins than in singletons. The higher frequency is probably due to an increased rate of malformations in monozygotic twins. Except for acardia and conjoined twins, the malformations seen are not specific for twins. Single umbilical arteries are more common in twins than in singleton fetuses and have been associated with IUGR, although the etiologic relationship has not been well established.[23] There is also a suggestion that midline birth defects are more common in twins. In the majority of cases congenital malformations are discordant (i.e., seen in only one of the fetuses). Concordance of malformations has been reported in varying frequencies ranging up to 18%.[22]

The entire range of chromosomal abnormalities can be seen in twins. With dizygotic twins usually only one of the twins is abnormal, whereas typically both are abnormal in monozygotic twinning. There have been some reports of discordant cases of genetic abnormalities with monozygotic twins, probably as a result of maldistribution of chromatin around the time of the twinning process. Trisomy 21 is not more commonly seen in twins, but there is some evidence that the incidence of Turner's and Klinefelter's syndromes is higher in twins.[22]

Abnormal intrauterine twin growth is also seen in twin-to-twin transfusion syndrome, in which blood flows from one fetus through vascular anastomoses in the placenta to its twin. These anastomoses are common in monochorionic placentas and can join artery to artery, vein to vein, or artery to vein. It is the artery-to-vein anastomosis that leads to a significant amount of blood transfusion from one fetus to the other. Acardia can be considered a severe form of twin-to-twin transfusion syndrome. One fetus develops without a heart; its tissues are perfused with blood pumped from its twin. There are two possible explanations for acardia: either the cardiac system never formed or was formed early in embryogenesis, only to later regress due to the hemodynamic influence of blood being transfused in from the other fetus. The "viable" twin has a significant risk for perinatal mortality, with congestive failure and growth retardation combining to adversely affect it.[24]

Typically, twin-to-twin transfusion syndrome is seen in the second trimester, with abnormalities of both fetuses. The donor fetus is found to be smaller, with a smaller placental mass and less amniotic fluid. Its twin is larger, with polyhydramnios (often acute), a larger placenta, and possibly hydrops. Measurement of serum protein levels obtained at birth suggests that the loss of blood from the donor fetus is not the only pathologic process present to explain its smaller growth. Newborn IgG levels—the result of transfer from maternal blood—have been found to be lower in donor twins than in recipients, whereas other fetal proteins—the result of fetal synthesis—are equal in the twins. This suggests that there is decreased transfer of nutrients from the mother to the donor fetus. Fetal outcome in twin-to-twin transfusion syndrome is poor, with mortality approaching 100% in some studies.

SIGNIFICANCE OF GROWTH RETARDATION IN TWINS

Of concern to the clinician is not that twin fetuses are smaller than singletons but the significance of this smaller weight on perinatal morbidity and mortality. In singletons there is a higher incidence of both morbidity and mortality with abnormal intrauterine growth. The data on the effects of growth retardation in twins is not so extensive, though we would predict findings similar to those in singletons.

It has been known for many years that low birth weight is the most significant factor for morbidity and mortality in twins. Most of the early studies did not distinguish between the relative effects of prematurity and growth retardation for their roles in both low birth weight and perinatal outcome. When birth weight is evaluated in relation to gestational age, prematurity has been found to be the most important factor for perinatal morbidity and mortality. IUGR, however, has been found to be the second most important factor overall for perinatal mortality, and is the primary cause of stillbirth.[25] As twin pregnancies progress into the third trimester, the role of growth retardation on outcome becomes more important and prematurity is less a factor.

Studies of intra-twin birth weight differences (discordancy) have also shown poorer outcome for the smaller twin. Babson et al.[26,27] examined various measures of intelligence in twin pairs where there was at least a 25% (arbitrarily selected) birth weight difference. In evaluation of these twin pairs (the entire group at an average follow-up of $8^1/_2$ years and the monozygotic twins again at an average of 18 years), higher IQ scores were found favoring the larger birth weight twin.[26,27] Other studies also report better outcomes in the larger twin.[28–31] Although one study found no outcome differences in discordant twins, the choice of a low value for discordance (15% birth weight difference) may have obscured twin differences.[32] The studies on discordant twins do not attempt to differentiate the various causes for the unequal weight (IUGR versus twin-to-twin transfusion).

Thus the findings of twin studies are similar to those in singletons. With IUGR the outcome can be adversely affected. Because of the high frequency of growth retardation in twins, close antenatal follow-up should be carried out in all twin pregnancies.

DIAGNOSIS OF IUGR IN TWINS

Ultrasonography has an integral role in the care of twin pregnancies because of its use for diagnosis of twins and serial evaluation of fetal health. Serial ultrasound studies should be obtained, starting at mid-gestation and repeated at 3- to 4-week intervals.

Early studies evaluating ultrasound examinations in twins concentrated on BPD, with varying results as to rate of growth when compared with singletons. More recently much has been published on the use of twin BPD differences (discordancy) to diagnose growth retardation. Here the larger twin serves as an internal control to assess the growth of the smaller infant. Care should be exercised in using the conclusions from these studies because of problems inherent in the use of BPD. Even in singletons, BPD has been found to be a poor predictor of birth weight. In twin gestations the accuracy of BPD is further compromised by the increased incidence of dolichocephaly due to fetal malposition. The use of BPD differences within a twin pregnancy would not be expected to enhance the detection of IUGR when both fetuses are affected, as in approximately 9.4% of twin pregnancies.

A summary of ultrasound studies on the usefulness of discordancy in predicting IUGR is given in Table 7–1. Cutoff points used for the definition of discordant BPDs and the sensitivity and false positive rates of these for IUGR are given. It is apparent from these studies that BPD differences are not accurate in diagnosing IUGR.

TABLE 7–1.
Prediction of IUGR by Difference in Biparietal Diameter

Source	BPD Cutoff for Discordancy (MM)	IUGR Sensitivity (%)	IUGR False-Positive (%)
Divers & Hemsell[33]	≥2	38.0	40.0
Houlton[34]	≥3	59.0	24.0
Erkkola et al.[35]	≥3	51.0	50.0
Houlton et al.[15]	≥3	35.0*	77.0
Barnea et al.[36]	≥3	55.5	73.0
Crane et al.[6]	≥5	100.0*	25.0
Leveno et al.[7]	≥5	54.0†	78.0
Houlton et al.[15]	≥5	9.0*	71.0
Houlton[34]	≥6	27.0	14.0
Erkkola et al.[35]	≥6	13.0	33.0
Barnea et al.[36]	≥6	55.5	37.5

*For >25% birth weight difference.
†For <1 SD below mean birth weight for twins.

TABLE 7–2.
Correlation of Twin Classification With Neonatal Morbidity

Classification System	Correlation (r^2) With Morbidity (%)	*P* Value
Gestational age	46.0	<0.001
Individual birth weight	6.2	<0.01
Discordancy	2.3	Not significant

More accurate results have been obtained using multiple ultrasound measurements. Evaluating various ultrasound parameters for their ability to predict IUGR in the smaller twin, Chitkara et al.[37] found abdominal circumference to be the most accurate single parameter. The most accurate overall parameter was estimated fetal weight, which was calculated from head and abdominal measurements.[37]

The physician should be cautious in using twin size differences as the best indication of IUGR. Neonatal data show that even twin birth weight differences are a poor predictor of growth retardation.[6] We evaluated data from our institution, and also believe discordancy is not the best means available to evaluate twins.[38] Twin birth weights were classified either in relation to the opposite twin (discordancy) or individually in relation to the singleton mean for gestational age. Both classifications were then correlated with a morbidity model constructed from a wide range of neonatal outcome variables. The effect of prematurity on morbidity was also tested. As shown in Table 7–2, prematurity very closely correlated with morbidity. Of the birth weight classifications, only individual weight in relation to gestational age correlated with morbidity. We find it questionable whether the use of twin size difference (discordancy) is the optimal means for evaluating twin pregnancies. Although the use of twin discordancy may be helpful in the case of a patient who registers for prenatal care late and has poor recollection of dates, we do not believe it the best use of the obtainable ultrasound data.

GUIDELINES FOR ANTENATAL CARE

Bed Rest

In an effort to improve perinatal outcome, bed rest, either at home or in the hospital, has long been recommended for women carrying twins. Reduction in maternal exertion and increase in uterine blood flow are possible mechanisms by which this therapy could be effective. Although extensively studied, the effectiveness of routine prophylactic bed rest has not been clearly established. Most studies on the effectiveness of bed rest are observational, without any prospective controlling and randomizing of patients and choice of therapy. It is difficult to draw statistically valid conclusions from such data. Table 7–3 shows the conclusions from recent reports on the effects

TABLE 7–3.
Effects of Bed Rest in Recent Studies

Source	Longer Duration of Pregnancy	Increased Birth Weight	Decreased Perinatal Mortality
Jeffrey et al[9]	−	+	+
Misenhimer and Kaltreider[39]	−	+	+
Weeks et al.[40]	−	−	−
Hawrylyshyn et al.[41]	+	−	−
Jouppila et al.[42]	−	−	+
Perrson et al.[43]	+	−	+
Sanders et al.[44]	−	−	−
Laursen[45]	+	+	+
Erkkola et al.[46]	−	−	+
Kappel et al.[47]	+	+	−

of bed rest in twin pregnancies; no uniform effect is supported by this data.

Although not fully supported by the literature, most reviews on twins state that bed rest probably does result in higher birth weight. Given the high frequency of growth retardation in twin gestations, we believe the recommendation of increased bed rest reasonable. Hospital bed rest is not absolutely necessary; good results with twin pregnancies have been obtained through the use of modified bed rest at home and with visits to a specialized outpatient clinic.[48] We recommend increased bed rest at home starting in mid-gestation.

Ultrasonography

We recommend serial ultrasound studies at intervals of 3 to 4 weeks beginning in mid-pregnancy. We believe it is best to evaluate the growth of each twin individually rather than in comparison with the other fetus. Also, because the birth weights in twins are lower than in singletons for pathologic not physiologic reasons, we recommend using singleton curves to assess growth. Growth curves specific for twins are less predictive of IUGR.

If IUGR is diagnosed, a more aggressive approach should be undertaken. We recommend hospital bed rest, although home bed rest may be an acceptable alternative in a supportive home environment. Attempts should be made to maximize nutrition and minimize smoking. At term, appropriate care would be delivery. In the preterm twin gestation with documented IUGR, management must reflect a balance between the morbidities from prematurity and growth retardation. Because of the wide range of pathologic disorders that can arise in twin pregnancies, no one single care plan can or should be outlined. Rather, the physician must be prepared to individualize therapy based on the specific details of each case.

Test of Fetal Well-Being

Antenatal assessment is begun in the mid–third trimester or earlier if indicated. The nonstress test is the first line of fetal assessment, but care must be taken to assure that each fetus is monitored. If there is any uncertainty as to whether each fetus was monitored, a biophysical profile should be performed.

Fetal Lung Maturity

If premature but elective delivery is contemplated, amniocentesis may be performed. Limited studies show that twins may have accelerated lung maturity compared with singleton fetuses. Both twins usually have similar lecithin/sphingomyelin (L/S) ratios, although if the sampling is done during labor twin A usually has the most advanced pulmonary status. IUGR in one twin has not been shown to result in significant twin L/S differences,[49–52] and in general sampling from only one sac is usually adequate to assess fetal lung maturity.

Current literature does not support a beneficial effect of antenatally administered steroids on the induction of fetal lung maturity. In the recent National Collaborative Study a beneficial effect was noted in singletons, with female fetuses responding better than male fetuses.[53] No effect was proved in twins, though the data suggested a trend similar to that in singletons. Female twins responded more favorably to steroids than male twins did, but this was not statistically significant. Cord blood levels of dexamethasone were found to be subtherapeutic in the treated twins,[54] suggesting that a different treatment regimen (higher doses or more frequent dosing) may result in significant improvement.

Route of Delivery

The appropriate route of delivery for twins is controversial.[13, 55] Most authors agree that when both twins are in the vertex position vaginal delivery is indicated. Recommendations are not so clear when one or both twins are in other than the vertex position. Appropriate considerations in determining delivery route include fetal positions, estimated fetal weights, availability of anesthesia, skill and comfort of the obstetrician with version and vaginal breech delivery, ability to monitor both fetuses during labor, and availability of ultrasonography during labor and delivery. Most articles on this subject view weight only in absolute terms and not in relation to gestational age. A growth-retarded fetus may not be able to tolerate the stress of labor. Also, twin B, when significantly larger than twin A, may sustain excessive trauma from breech extraction.

There is no one correct way for twins to be delivered. Given the current medicolegal constraints on obstetrical practice, many physicians are seeking standards to guide their actions. We do not believe that it is appropriate to set rigid guidelines for the delivery of twins. Choice of the route of delivery must be individualized for each pregnancy.

SUMMARY

In this chapter the role of intrauterine growth retardation in twin pregnancies has been reviewed. This chapter should not be separated, at least conceptually, from the rest of the book. The factors that play a role in singleton growth are also important in twin growth. The considerations on the part of the obstetrician faced with growth retardation in twins are similar to those in singleton gestations, with the added role of factors specific for twins (e.g., twin-to-twin transfusion). Anticipation along with appropriate diagnostic testing and individualized therapeutic actions should be undertaken to maximize perinatal outcome.

REFERENCES

1. McKeown T, Record RG: Observations on fetal growth in multiple pregnancies in man. *J Endocrinol* 1952; 8:386.
2. Daw E, Walker J: Growth differences in twin pregnancy. *Br J Clin Pract* 1975; 29:150.
3. Leroy B, Lefort F, Neveu P, et al: Intrauterine growth charts for twin fetuses. *Acta Genet Med Gemellol (Roma)* 1982; 31:199.
4. Bleker OP, Kloosterman GJ, Huidekoper BL, et al: Intrauterine growth of twins as estimates from birth weight and the fetal biparietal diameter. *Eur J Obstet Gynecol Reprod Biol* 1977; 7:85.
5. Bleker OP, Breur W, Huidekoper BL: A study of birth weight, placental weight and mortality of twins as compared to singletons. *Br J Obstet Gynaecol* 1979; 86:111.
6. Crane JP, Tomich PG, Kopta M: Ultrasonic growth patterns in normal and discordant twins. *Obstet Gynecol* 1980; 55:678.
7. Leveno KJ, Santos-Ramos R, Duenhoelter JH: Sonar cephalometry in twins: A table of biparietal diameters for normal twin fetuses and a comparison with singletons. *Am J Obstet Gynecol* 1979; 135:727.
8. O'Brien WF, Knuppel RA, Scerbo JC, et al: Birth weight in twins: An analysis of discordancy and growth retardation. *Obstet Gynecol* 1980; 67:43.
9. Jeffrey RL, Bowes WA, Delaney JJ: Role of bed rest in twin gestation. *Obstet Gynecol* 1974; 43:822.
10. Chervenak FA, Youcha S, Johnson RE, et al: Twin gestation: Antenatal diagnosis and perinatal outcome in 385 consecutive pregnancies. *J Reprod Med* 1984; 29:727.
11. Ho SK, Wu PYK: Perinatal factors and neonatal morbidity in twin pregnancy. *Am J Obstet Gynecol* 1975; 122:979.

12. Koivisto M, Jouppila P, Kauppila A, et al: Twin pregnancy: Neonatal morbidity and mortality. *Acta Obstet Gynecol Scand* [Suppl] 1975; 44:21.
13. Cetrulo CL: The controversy of mode of delivery in twins: The intrapartum management of twin gestation (part I). *Semin Perinatol* 1986; 10:39.
14. Hemon D, Berger C, Lazar P: Maternal factors associated with small-for-dateness among twins. *Acta Genet Med Gemellol (Roma)* 1982; 31:241.
15. Houlton MCC, Marivate M, Philpott RH: The prediction of fetal growth retardation in twin pregnancy. *Br J Obstet Gynaecol* 1982; 88:264.
16. Corney G, Robson EB, Strong SJ: The effect of zygosity on the birth weight of twins. *Ann Hum Genet* 1972; 36:45.
17. Bjoro K Jr, Bjoro K: Disturbed intrauterine growth in twins: Etiological aspects. *Acta Genet Med Gemellol (Roma)* 1985; 34:73.
18. Wharton B, Edwards JH, Cameron AH: Monoamniotic twins. *J Obstet Gynaec Br Commonw* 1968; 75:158.
19. Tarkowski AK: Experiments on the development of isolated blastomeres of mouse eggs. *Nature* 1959; 184:1286.
20. Bowman P, McLaren A: Viability and growth of mouse embryos after in vitro culture and fusion. *J Embryol Exp Morphol* 1970; 23:693.
21. Wilson RS: Twin growth: Initial deficit, recovery, and trends in concordance from birth to nine years. *Ann Hum Biol* 1979; 6:205.
22. Little J, Bryan E: Congenital anomalies in twins. *Semin Perinatol* 1986; 10:50.
23. Heifetz SA: Single umbilical artery: A statistical analysis of 237 autopsy cases and review of the literature. *Perspect Pediatr Pathol* 1984; 8:345.
24. Van Allen MI, Smith DW, Shepard TH: Twin reversed arterial perfusion (TRAP) sequence: A study of 14 twin pregnancies with acardius. *Semin Perinatol* 1983; 7:285.
25. Manlan G, Scott KE: Contribution of twin pregnancy to perinatal mortality and fetal growth retardation: Reversal of growth retardation after birth. *Can Med Assoc J* 1978; 118:365.
26. Babson G, Kangas J, Young N, et al: Growth and development of twins of dissimilar size at birth. *Pediatrics* 1964; 33:327.
27. Babson SG, Phillips DS: Growth and development of twins dissimilar in size at birth. *N Engl J Med* 1973; 289:937.
28. Drillien CM: The incidence of mental and physical handicaps in school-age children of very low birth weight. *Pediatrics* 1966; 27:452.
29. Churchill JA: The relationship between intelligence and birth weight in twins. *Neurology* 1985; 15:341.
30. Drillien CM: The small-for-date infant: Etiology and prognosis. *Pediatr Clin North Am* 1970; 17:9.
31. Kaelber CT, Pugh TF: Influence of intrauterine relations on the intelligence of twins. *N Engl J Med* 1969; 280:1030.
32. Fujikura T, Froehlich LA: Mental and motor development in monozygotic cotwins with dissimilar birth weights. *Pediatrics* 1974; 53:884.
33. Divers WA, Hemsell DL: The use of ultrasound in multiple gestations. *Obstet Gynecol* 1979; 53:500.
34. Houlton MC: Divergent biparietal diameter growth rates in twin pregnancies. *Obstet Gynecol* 1977; 49:542.

35. Erkkola R, Ala-Mello S, Piiroinen O: Growth discordancy in twin pregnancies: A risk factor not detected by measurements of biparietal diameter. *Obstet Gynecol* 1985; 66:203.
36. Barnea ER, Romero R, Scott D, et al: The value of biparietal diameter and abdominal perimeter in the diagnosis of growth retardation in twin gestation. *Am J Perinatol* 1985; 2:221.
37. Chitkara U, Berkowitz GS, Levine R, et al: Twin pregnancy: Routine use of ultrasound examinations in the prenatal diagnosis of intrauterine growth retardation and discordant growth. *Perinatol* 1985; 2:49.
38. Bronsteen R, Goyert G, Bottoms S: Prediction of neonatal morbidity in twins: IUGR vs. discordancy. Presented at Society of Perinatal Obstetricians, Lake Buena Vista, Fla, 1987.
39. Misenhimer HR, Kaltreider DR: Effects of decreased prenatal activity in patients with twin pregnancy. *Obstet Gynecol* 1978; 51:692.
40. Weeks ARL, Menzies DN, DeBoer CH: The relative efficacy of bed rest, cervical suture, and no treatment in the management of twin pregnancy. *Br J Obstet Gynaecol* 1977; 84:161.
41. Hawrylyshyn PA, Barkin M, Bernstein A, et al: Twin pregnancies—A continuing perinatal challenge. *Obstet Gynecol* 1982; 59:463.
42. Jouppila P, Kauppila A, Koivisto M, et al: Twin pregnancy: The role of active management during pregnancy and delivery. *Acta Obstet Gynecol Scand* 1975; 44:13.
43. Perrson PH, Grennert L, Gennser G, et al: On improved outcome of twin pregnancies. *Acta Obstet Gynecol Scand* 1979; 58:3.
44. Sanders MC, Dick JS, Brown IM, et al: The effects of hospital admission for bed rest on the duration of twin pregnancy: A randomized trial. Lancet 1985; 2:793.
45. Laursen B: Twin pregnancy: The value of prophylactic rest in bed and the risks involved. *Acta Obstet Gynecol Scand* 1973; 52:367.
46. Erkkola R, Ala-Mello S, Kero P, et al: Fetal growth and perinatal mortality in twin pregnancy. *Int J Gynaecol Obstet* 1985; 23:115.
47. Kappel B, Hansen KB, Moller J, et al: Bed rest in twin pregnancy. *Acta Genet Med Gemellol (Roma)* 1985; 34:67.
48. O'Connor MC, Arias E, Royston JP, et al: The merits of special antenatal care for twin pregnancies. *Br J Obstet Gynaecol* 1981; 88:22.
49. Spellacy WN, Cruz AC, Buhi WC, et al: Amniotic fluid L/S ratio in twin gestation. *Obstet Gynecol* 1977; 50:68.
50. Norman RJ, Joubert SM, Marivate M: Amniotic fluid phospholipids and glucocorticoids in multiple pregnancies. *Br J Obstet Gynaecol* 1983; 90:51.
51. Sims CD, Cowan DB, Parkinson CE: The lecithin sphingomyelin (L/S) ratio in twin pregnancies. *Br J Obstet Gynaecol* 1976; 83:447.
52. Leveno KJ, Quirk JG, Whalley PJ, et al: Fetal lung maturation in twin gestation. *Am J Obstet Gynecol* 1984; 148:405.
53. *Prevention of Respiratory Distress: Effect of Antenatal Dexamethasone Administration.* US Department of Health and Human Services, NIH Publication No 85-2695, August 1985.
54. Burkett G, Bauer C, Morrison SC, et al: Effect of prenatal dexamethasone administration on prevention of respiratory distress syndrome in twin pregnancies. *J Perinatol* 1986; 6:305.

55. Chervenak FA: The controversy of mode of delivery in twins: The intrapartum management of twin gestation (part II). *Semin Perinatol* 1986; 10:44.

PART IV

Diagnostic Approaches

8

The Role of Clinical Determinants in Predicting Intrauterine Growth Retardation

Robert A. Welch, M.D.
Honor M. Wolfe, M.D.
Robert J. Sokol, M.D.

The timely diagnosis of intrauterine growth retardation (IUGR) logically should occur during the course of good prenatal care. Although this is hypothetically the case, a precise way to accurately diagnose IUGR remains elusive despite the many other landmark achievements in obstetrical diagnosis in recent years. Brown et al.[1] recently concluded that normal ultrasound findings are highly predictive of appropriately grown neonates. But it appears that even ultrasonography is unreliable in identifying the fetus with IUGR, with accuracy at 65% at best.

A large proportion of fetuses with IUGR have subsequent neonatal morbidity and a higher prevalence of childhood neurobehavioral abnormalities.[2–4] They are four to eight times more susceptible to perinatal mortality (e.g., intrapartum fetal death, stillbirth) than are normally grown infants.[5] Frequently IUGR is undiagnosed because maternal entry into the prenatal health care system is late or because of a low level of suspicion on the part of the clinician.

This chapter is written specifically to make the clinician "think IUGR" in his or her daily encounter with patients. The clinical risk factors for IUGR are reviewed. Laborious detail about the etiology of IUGR is omitted because

TABLE 8–1.
Risk Factors for IUGR

Socioeconomic	Obstetrical
Young age	Primigravid
Unmarried	Previous SGA infant
Poor nutrition	Previous spontaneous abortion
Substance abuse (tobacco, alcohol, or drugs)	Previous stillbirth
Medical conditions	Pregnancy complications
Essential hypertension	Preeclampsia
Kidney disease	Third-trimester bleeding disorders
Chronic anemia	Preterm labor
Autoimmune disease	Preterm premature rupture of membranes
Diabetes > class B	Poor maternal weight gain
	Poor uterine fundal growth
	Multiple gestation
Maternal infections	Genetic disorders
Listeriosis	Trisomies 13, 18, 21
Tuberculosis	Turner's syndrome
Syphilis	Neural tube defects
TORCH infections	Congenital heart defects
Malaria	

clinically we generally focus on whether IUGR is present rather than why. Key aspects of these risk factors are highlighted in the text and summarized in Table 8–1. We conclude with our own observations about predicting IUGR on a clinical basis.

SOCIOECONOMIC RISKS FOR IUGR

Socioeconomic status is difficult to completely assess as a cause of IUGR because of the complexity of the factors involved. An inherent pitfall for the physician is that traditional training is heavily directed at diagnosing disease processes while ignoring the patient's socioeconomic situation. Thus consideration of the mother's socioeconomic status may be difficult or easily overlooked at the first obstetric visit. Frequently the patient is interviewed by a nonmedical office employee (e.g., receptionist, biller), and her socioeconomic status never reaches the attention of the clinician. Socioeconomic status may also relate to maternal health practices and may provide the clinician with invaluable leads in predicting IUGR.

The effects of socioeconomic status are approached by subdividing the topic into some key areas: (1) nutrition, (2) adverse habits (substance use or abuse), (3) the working mother, and (4) exercise and concerns about body image during pregnancy.

Nutrition

The cause of abnormal fetal growth based on socioeconomic group appears to be multifaceted. Effects of several related factors (e.g., age, parity, nutrition) on fetal growth are difficult to differentiate by socioeconomic class. Though of uncertain applicability in humans, maternal protein and calorie restriction in animals adversely affects fetal growth.[6] Conversely, we often assume that patients from higher socioeconomic groups consume a balanced diet; in practice this group may be more likely to have food fetishes ("vegan" diet) or follow fad diets.

Regardless of socioeconomic status, several clinical determinants suggest abnormal maternal nutritional habits that may be associated with IUGR. Iron (microcytic, hypochromic indices) or folate (macrocytic, hypochromic indices) deficiency anemia may be detected during initial prenatal screening. Failure to gain weight in the second trimester also deserves close scrutiny. Persistent spilling of urinary ketones in combination with anemia or failure to gain weight is highly suggestive of modified starvation. Any combination of these factors merits dietary consultation and review of maternal eating habits.

Adverse Habits (Substance Use or Abuse)

Miller and Merritt[7] noted that mothers of low socioeconomic status are twice as likely as mothers of high socioeconomic status to engage in adverse habits (e.g., use of tobacco, alcohol, or drugs). These practices are not always restricted by maternal socioeconomic group. For several years it has been known that maternal cigarette smoking is related to low birth weight,[8] an effect possibly mediated by increased carboxyhemoglobin[9] or thiocyanate levels.[10,11] Bottoms et al.[12] have also demonstrated high thiocyanate levels in maternal and fetal serum from pregnancies exposed to passive smoking.

Maternal alcohol consumption, a factor that may be difficult to elicit from maternal history,[13] is also related to IUGR. A study of alcoholism by Sokol et al.[14] found that "clinicians are continuing to miss the diagnosis in at least three of every four alcohol-abusing patients. It is unlikely that there is any other obstetric diagnosis that is missed as often." Two percent to 13% of North American women drink excessively during pregnancy.[15]

Experimentation leading to frequent usage or addiction to other drugs of abuse must also be sought. The user may look physically exhausted; pupils may be dilated or constricted; signs of the pregnancy may not coincide with the stated gestational age; there may be track marks, abscesses, or edema of the upper or lower extremities; the nasal mucosa may be inflamed or indurated; or the patient may seem disoriented.[16] Preliminary data from the University of Michigan suggest that as many as 30% of college graduates have tried cocaine and other highly addictive substances. Infants delivered of mothers who have used cocaine during pregnancy tend to be shorter and to have lower birth weight and smaller head circumference than infants delivered of drug-free women. Narcotic addition is a well-known cause of IUGR.[17]

The Working Mother

Approximately 50% of American households are supported by both parents working outside of the home. Consequently, working women constitute a significant proportion of many office practices, yet research into the potential effects of the work environment on pregnancy has lagged. Often gravidas are required to stand for long periods, forego sleep in order to "punch the clock" on time, or are exposured to noxious agents (e.g., benzene) that have potential to affect fetal growth. The impact of these factors on fetal growth has not been conclusively established in the current literature.

Alegre et al.[18] showed reduced mean fetal weight in both primigravidas and multigravidas who worked, compared with a nonworking cohort. Grunebaum et al.[19] recently presented their findings regarding the effects of obstetric residency, a physically demanding type of work, on fetal growth. Firstborn infants delivered during residency were found to be significantly smaller than firstborn infants delivered before residency. The low birth weight rate was also higher during residency than before or after. The most striking finding was that infants born during residency were 7.5 times more likely to be growth retarded than those born before or after residency.

Others have shown no association between work activity and the incidence of IUGR. In contrast to the studies cited above, Meyer and Daling[20] stratified women in Washington by work activity levels and found no effect on the incidence of low birth weight. Overall, these initial studies of working mothers and their pregnancy outcomes serve as a background for further investigation into specific factors in the work place. With the exclusion of exposure to the most dangerous of work environments (e.g., exposure to radiation), a categorical recommendation about the safety of working during pregnancy and potential effects on fetal growth cannot be made.

We generally recommend that patients in clerical or sales jobs work until 2 weeks before the expected date of confinement. Patients who stand for long periods (e.g., assembly line workers) often can be transferred to more sedentary positions. If diminished fetal growth is suspected during the course of prenatal care based on clinical or ultrasound criterion, we recommend a medical leave of absence. Consideration of the patient's occupation is often overlooked by obstetrical care providers.

Exercise and Concerns About Body Image During Pregnancy

Acceptance of the concept that one can modify his or her health destiny by "eating right," not smoking, and regular exercise may prove to be as significant to societal health today as the recognition of the basic food groups and improved hygiene were to the previous generation. Some gravidas, however, may become obsessed with strenuous exercise at the expense of the pregnancy. Similar to studies on work activity in pregnancy, studies focusing on the effects of exercise in pregnancy on fetal growth report contrasting findings.[21–23]

There is little doubt that exercise to the extent of endurance training shortens gestation and causes low birth weight.[21] Limited exercise has not been shown to adversely affect fetal growth. Conversely, there is no evidence to support the popular notion that regular exercise will improve the outcome of pregnancy. The fetal response to vigorous maternal exercise may include episodes of bradycardia, but the actual incidence and significance are unknown.[23] Such bradycardia could represent brief periods of fetal asphyxia.

As with work activity, the effect of maternal exercise on fetal growth deserves ongoing scrutiny during the course of routine prenatal care. We recommend the American College of Obstetricians and Gynecologists *Pregnancy and Postnatal Exercise Programs*[24] to patients who inquire about exercise routines during pregnancy. This series is provided in video, tape, and record formats and is suited to a broad section of the population.

RISKS FOR IUGR IN THE OBSTETRIC HISTORY

The history of a previous small for gestational age (SGA) infant is among the most significant risks for growth retardation in subsequent pregnancies. The recurrence risk for SGA in the overall obstetric population, even in the absence of other pregnancy complications, has been noted to be as high as 25%.[25,26] Patterson et al.[27] reported that the combination of a history of a previous SGA neonate and an additional complication in the current pregnancy act synergistically to increase the risk for growth retardation to a level higher than that attributable to either risk factor alone.

It is often difficult to determine from the maternal history whether a previous newborn was growth retarded, premature, or both. Because the risk factors and morbidity preceding IUGR are different from those preceding prematurity, determining whether the previous infant was growth retarded is worthwhile. This may sometimes be performed by including both the birth weight and the gestational age in the medical record. Quick referral to a newborn growth chart will indicate whether the previous newborn's birth weight was in the lower 10th percentile for gestational age (SGA). When the patient is unable to provide gestational age information about the newborn, she may remember the estimated date of confinement, thus allowing calculation of the gestational age at the time of delivery. This provides a rough estimate about the past history of IUGR and may be the basis for a clinical suspicion of the likelihood of IUGR in the present pregnancy.

RISKS ASSOCIATED WITH MATERNAL MEDICAL CONDITIONS

When the pregnancy is complicated by an underlying maternal medical condition (e.g., hypertension), the risk for IUGR is exceptionally high. This relates partially to the physiologic stresses on the fetus caused by the vascular spasms, microvascular thrombi, and reduced uterine perfusion associated with these disorders. Prediction of IUGR by the clinician on purely clinical grounds may be possible if the maternal illness is severe.

These highly selected, or bias, groups form the basis for several ultrasound studies using amniotic fluid volume to predict IUGR.[28] Villar et al.[4] remind us that the sensitivity and specificity of any test depend on the prevalence of the condition in the population under consideration. Thus many ultrasound studies evaluating fetal growth may be subject to selection bias introduced by clinicians who already have predicted IUGR based on substantial clinical evidence. This has caused skepticism among some that clinical prediction may be comparable to ultrasound prediction of IUGR. In the select case of severe maternal illness this may be so, but as we will demonstrate later, this opinion does not appear to be justified in the majority of circumstances.

Space does not permit us to summarize all of the maternal medical disorders related to IUGR. A few simple questions about the pathophysiologic mechanisms of the underlying disease help to foster consideration of their metabolic impact on fetal growth.

Does the Disease Disturb Maternal Absorption or Cause Loss of Proteins?—Although various degrees of hyperemesis gravidarum may occur early in pregnancy, it is infrequent that it causes prolonged, decreased maternal protein absorption significant enough to be associated with IUGR. However, a history of protein-wasting enteropathies, ulcerative colitis, chronic pancreatitis, and similar more severe gastrointestinal disorders are definite risks for IUGR. In addition, one of the major effects of severe kidney disease on pregnancy is protein loss in the urine, resulting in IUGR.[29]

Does the Disease Affect Materno-fetal Metabolism?—If the disease affects blood flow to or from the placenta, as in cyanotic maternal cardiac disease or severe anemia, essential nutrient and oxygen exchange across the placenta may be decreased to such an extent that IUGR results.

Does the Disease Affect Maternal Blood Vessels?—Maternal vascular disease, whether due to renal disease, essential or pregnancy-induced hypertension, or diabetes, appears to be the single most common denominator in the cause of IUGR.[30] Visser et al.[31] found evidence of IUGR in as many as 50% of gestations associated with severe hypertensive disorders. Fetal growth appeared to be retarded at an earlier gestational age than with other causes of IUGR.

INCIPIENT RISKS FOR IUGR

Prenatal events affecting fetal growth may be as dramatic as the hemorrhaging placenta previa or as subtle as poor progression of uterine fundal growth. They are perhaps best considered by reviewing routine prenatal care and then focusing more specifically on individual events.

The Benefits of Prenatal Care in Predicting IUGR

Although its value has been questioned,[32] routine prenatal care provides an opportunity for early recognition of developing complications that may affect fetal growth. After the first visit, the routine prenatal visit consists of a few simple measures of maternal and fetal well-being (e.g., blood pressure, weight gain, McDonald's measurement of uterine fundus growth, assessment of fetal lie and fetal heart tones, and dipstick urinalysis). Suspect or abnormal trends in these values probably serve their greatest purpose by prompting more thorough evaluation of fetal growth (e.g., ultrasound studies).

McDonald's measurement of symphysis-fundus distance, serves as a reference for fetal growth and confirmation of gestational age. Classically, fundal height between 18 and 38 weeks corresponds on a weeks per centimeter basis. The value of this measurement remains controversial.[33] Deviation from what is expected for gestational age still acts as an early predictor of IUGR and should prompt further investigation of fetal growth in most clinical settings.

Prenatal care is not complete without the ready availability of genetic diagnosis. As demonstrated in Table 8–1, a host of genetic disorders may account for IUGR. The presence of a genetic disorder may alter subsequent clinical management, and should be considered if IUGR is suspected.

The Role of Prenatal Care in Confirming Dates

Reliable knowledge of the duration of pregnancy prior to birth is crucial and forms the basis for the diagnosis of IUGR. Apart from its value in recognizing developing risks, routine prenatal care is beneficial in establishing gestational age. A reliable last menstrual period (i.e., of normal character, of certain date, and in a patient with regular menses) is the most accurate clinical estimator of gestational age.[34] Results of a pregnancy test, first audible fetal heart tones by fetoscope, or quickening documented early in the pregnancy may be extremely useful in confirming historical dating parameters.

Developing Complications and Their Relationship to Fetal Growth

Evidence suggests that the development of complications in an otherwise normal pregnancy may be related to abnormal fetal growth. Several investigators have suggested the relationship of IUGR to preterm premature rupture of the membranes (PROM).[35] It seems logical that the abnormally grown fetus may also have abnormal fetal membranes more susceptible to early rupture. Abnormal fetal growth may also explain the confusion in ultrasound measurements frequently seen in pregnancies with preterm PROM.[36] Previously, low fetal measurements in preterm pregnancies complicated by PROM were thought to be secondary to fetal compression or less than optimal ultrasound resolution. Recent investigations suggest that they may be the result of diminished fetal growth associated with rupture of the fetal membranes. This poses the problem of underestimating the gestational age in these fetuses, leading to inappropriate treatment decisions. IUGR is also known to be associated with preterm labor and may be responsible for enhanced lung maturity in some cases, as opposed to the stress of premature labor.

THE PREGNANCY AT RISK FOR IUGR

Uniform Perinatal Risk Scoring

It is impossible to consider all risk factors in every patient at each prenatal visit. Several investigators have simplified the process by developing risk assessment tools aimed at predicting later pregnancy complications.[37, 39] These risk assessment forms (e.g., POPRAS or Hollister) help to organize the prenatal data and, with experience, greatly simplify appropriate documentation of key risk factors. They appear to increase the odds of clinically identifying the woman at risk for delivering an SGA infant.

Typical Pregnancy at Risk for IUGR

Several studies[25, 40–42] published since 1970 have attempted to evaluate clinical risk factors associated with delivery of an SGA infant and to express the results in statistical models. Reasonably consistent clinical risks associated with IUGR are common in these studies. Typically these factors include small maternal size, youth or primiparity, birth of a previous low birth weight infant, hypertension, preeclampsia, and cigarette smoking. Given the consistency with which these factors show up in different studies of different populations from different periods in different countries, their presence in a pregnancy should immediately increase the clinician's index of suspicion for IUGR.

CLINICAL INABILITY TO PREDICT IUGR

The Performance of Clinical Risk Factors in the Prediction of IUGR

Although many clinical risk factors are associated with IUGR, their usefulness in actually predicting IUGR, except in the most extreme cases, appears limited. Perinatal risk scoring schemes, though appealing to many clinicians and useful for tracking information, are similarly limited because they rely on these clinical factors. Adelstein and Fedrick[43] demonstrated that based on their scoring system nearly half of the SGA infants at term were unsuspected. In a hypothetical 10,000 first pregnancies, 1,930 (20%) women would be classified as at high risk. Of these, only 153 women would be expected to deliver an SGA infant at term.

Sokol et al.[44] developed a model for IUGR based on relative risk factors including fundal growth measurements in a data set consisting of 2,310 pregnancies (Table 8–2). When this model was applied to an additional 3,105 term pregnancies including 514 (9.5%) SGA infants, fewer than 40% of IUGR pregnancies were predicted. The 20% of the sample considered at greatest risk included only 55% of the SGA infants. They concluded that nearly 50% of pregnancies complicated by IUGR could not possibly be identified on the basis of clinical risk alone, because they occurred in the low-risk group. Nonetheless, when the listed risks were present singly or in combination, IUGR was considerably more likely.

Combining Clinical Risks With Ultrasound: The Two-Step Approach

Inasmuch as the ability to predict an SGA infant on the basis of clinical risk assessment alone appears to be severely limited, a two-step approach to the diagnosis has been advocated. In the first screening step maternal risk

TABLE 8–2.
Clinical Rule for IUGR Detection

Risk*	Prevalence (%)	Relative Risk (X)
No previous non-LBW infants	47.2	1.7
Black race	50.7	2.3
Height <62 inches	19.6	1.5
Weight <100 lb	3.8	2.4
Narcotic abuse	0.8	2.1
Cigarettes >1 pack/day	42.6	1.6
Hobel antenatal risk score >20	49.9	1.3
Systolic BP >160	1.3	1.6

*Note: These independent risks are adjusted for other present risks. They are minimally additive. Thus for a black multigravida who smokes and who has had one or more infants with low birth weight, risk for the birth of an SGA infant would be more than 50%

factors are identified and fundal height is measured; in the second step those fetuses with suspected IUGR are examined by ultrasound.[45,46]

In a recent review Villar and Belizan[47] noted that as many as 73% of fetuses with IUGR could be predicted using this technique. However, they emphasized that clinicians need to be trained to recognize perinatal risk factors, appropriately measure uterine fundal growth, and monitor maternal weight gain, and to plot these findings on legible flow curves. (This is described in detail in Chapter 9.) Others[43,44] have been less optimistic about the use of clinical factors for screening. They suggest that, at best, 50% of fetuses with IUGR will be identified in any effort based on clinical factors. The problem rests with "undersensitivity," that is, missing the cases without clinical risk factors. Given the value of prenatal detection of IUGR, this may be a cogent argument in favor of extended use of prenatal sonography.

CONCLUSION

Clinical risks alone do not appear adequate to consistently predict IUGR. When applied in an optimal manner or in the two-step approach, it appears that the best that can be expected is diagnosis of between 50% and 73% of cases. It may be possible for clinicians to improve their individual performances by diligent use of prenatal risk scoring schemes and by plotting maternal weight gain and uterine fundal growth. However, it appears that even these efforts will miss a significant number of fetuses with IUGR. Because of the perinatal risk associated with IUGR, liberal use of ultrasound examination appears to be justified.

REFERENCES

1. Brown HL, Miller JM, Gabert HA, et al: Ultrasonic recognition of the small-for-gestational age fetus. *Obstet Gynecol* 1987; 69:631.
2. Low JA, Galbraith RS, Muri D, et al: Intrauterine growth retardation: A preliminary report of long-term morbidity. *Am J Obstet Gynecol* 1978; 130:534.
3. Fancourt R, Campbell S, Harvey D, et al: Follow-up study of small-for-dates-babies. *Br Med J* 1976; 1:1435.
4. Villar J, Belizan JM, Spalding J, et al: Postnatal growth of intrauterine growth retarded infants. *Early Hum Dev* 1982; 6:165.
5. Koops BL, Morgan LJ, Battaglia FC: Neonatal mortality risk in relation to birth weight and gestational age: Update. *J Pediatr* 1982; 101:969.
6. Brasel JA, Winick M: Maternal nutrition and prenatal growth: Experimental studies of effects of maternal undernutrition on fetal and placental growth. *Arch Dis Child* 1972; 47:479.
7. Miller HC, Merritt TA: *Fetal Growth in Humans*. Chicago, Year Book Medical Publishers, 1979.

8. Simpson WJ: A preliminary report on cigarette smoking and the incidence of prematurity. *Am J Obstet Gynecol* 1957; 73:808.
9. Cole PV, Hawkins LH, Robert D: Smoking during pregnancy and its effects on the fetus. *J Obstet Gynaecol Br Commonw* 1972; 79:782.
10. Meberg A, Sande H, Foss OP, et al: Smoking during pregnancy—Effects on the fetus and on thiocyanate levels in mother and baby. *Acta Paediatr Scand* 1979, 68:547.
11. Andrews J: Thiocyanate and smoking in pregnancy. *J Obstet Gynaecol Br Commonw* 1973; 80:810.
12. Bottoms SF, Kuhnert BR, Kuhnert PM, et al: Maternal passive smoking and fetal serum thiocyanate levels. *Am J Obstet Gynecol* 1982; 144:787.
13. Sokol RJ: Avoiding alcohol related birth defects. *Contemp Obstet Gynecol* 1986; 27:27.
14. Sokol RJ, Miller SI, Martier S: Preventing Fetal Alcohol Effects: A Practical Guide for OB/GYN Physicians and Nurses. Rockville, Md, National Institute on Alcohol Abuse and Alcoholism, 1981.
15. Sokol RJ, Miller SI, Reed G: Alcohol abuse during pregnancy: An epidemiologic study. *Alcoholism* (NY) 1980; 4:135.
16. Chasnoff IJ: Perinatal effects of cocaine. *Contemp Obstet Gynecol* 1987; 29:163.
17. Connaughton J, Reeser D, Schut J, et al: Perinatal addictions: Outcome and management. *Am J Obstet Gynecol* 1977; 129:679.
18. Alegre A, Rodriguez-Escudero FJ, Cruz E, et al: Influence of work during pregnancy on fetal weight. *J Reprod Med* 1984; 29:334.
19. Grunebaum A, Blake D, Minkoff H: Pregnancy outcome among female obstetricians: The relationship of residency to infant's birthweight, in *Proceedings of the Sixth Annual Meeting of the Society of Perinatal Obstetricians*, Las Vegas, Jan 30–Feb 1, 1986.
20. Meyer BA, Daling JR: Activity level of mother's usual occupation and low infant birth weight. *J Occup Med* 1985; 11:841.
21. Clapp JF, Dickstein S: Endurance exercise and pregnancy outcome. *Med Sci Sports Exerc* 1984; 16:556.
22. Gorski J: Exercise during pregnancy: Maternal and fetal response. A brief review. *Med Sci Sports Exerc* 1985; 17:407.
23. Lotgering FK, Gilbert RD, Longo LD: Maternal and fetal response to exercise during pregnancy. *Physiol Rev* 1985; 65:1.
24. *ACOG Pregnancy and Postnatal Exercise Programs.* East Washington, DC, The American College of Obstetricians and Gynecologists.
25. Hedberg E, and Holmdahl K: On relationship between maternal health and intrauterine growth of the foetus. *Acta Obstet Gynecol Scand* 1970; 49:225.
26. Wolfe HM, Gross TL, Sokol RJ: Recurrent small for gestational age birth: Perinatal risks and outcomes. *Am J Obstet Gynecol* 1987; 157:288.
27. Patterson RM, Gibbs CE, Wood RC: Birth weight percentile in perinatal outcome: Recurrence of intrauterine growth retardation. *Obstet Gynecol* 1986; 68:464.
28. Hoddick WK, Callen PW, Filly RA, et al: Ultrasonographic determination of qualitative amniotic fluid volume in intrauterine growth retardation: Reassessment of the 1 cm rule. *Am J Obstet Gynecol* 1984; 149:758.

29. Welch RA, Evans MI, Sokol RJ: Maternal and fetal complications, in Peyreya JL: *Complications of Organ Transplantation*. New York, Marcel Dekker, 1987.
30. Keirse MJNC: Aetiology of intrauterine growth retardation, in van Assche, FA, Robertson WB, Renaer M, *Fetal Growth Retardation*. Edinburgh, Churchill Livingstone, 1981, p 37.
31. Visser GHA, Huisman A, Saathof PWF, et al: Early fetal growth retardation: Obstetric background and recurrence rate. *Obstet Gynecol* 1986; 67:40.
32. Hall M, Chang PK, MacGilluray I: Is routine antenatal care worthwhile? *Lancet* 1980; 2:78.
33. Bagger PV, Eriksen PS, Secher NJ, et al: The precision and accuracy of symphysis-fundus distance measurements during pregnancy. *Acta Obstet Gynecol Scand* 1985; 64:371.
34. Hertz RH, Sokol RJ, Knoke JD, et al: Clinical estimation of gestational age: Rules for avoiding preterm delivery. *Am J Obstet Gynecol* 1978; 131:395.
35. Tamura RK, Sabbagha RE, Depp R, et al: Diminished growth in fetuses born preterm after spontaneous labor or rupture of membranes. *Am J Obstet Gynecol* 1984; 148:1105.
36. Bottoms SF, Welch RA, Zador IE, et al: Clinical interpretation of ultrasound measurements in preterm pregnancies with premature rupture of the membranes. *Obstet Gynecol* 1987; 69:358.
37. Nesbitt RE, Aubry RH: High-risk obstetrics. II: Value of semiobjective grading system in identifying the vulnerable groups. *Am J Obstet Gynecol* 1969; 103:972.
38. Hobel CH, Hyvarinen MA, Okada DM, et al: Prenatal and intrapartum high risk screen. 1: Prediction of the high risk neonate. *Am J Obstet Gynecol* 1973; 117:1.
39. Sokol RJ, Rosen MG, Stojkon J, et al: Clinical application of high risk scoring on an obstetrical service. *Am J Obstet Gynecol* 1977; 128:652.
40. Low JA, Galbraith RS: Pregnancy characteristics of intrauterine growth retardation. *Obstet Gynecol* 1974; 44:122.
41. Fedrick J, Adelstein P: Factors associated with low birthweight of infants delivered at term. *Br J Obstet Gynaecol* 1978; 85:1.
42. Wennergren M, Karlsson K: A scoring system for antenatal identification of fetal growth retardation. *Br J Obstet Gynaecol* 1982; 89:520.
43. Adelstein P, Fedrick J: Antenatal identification of women at increased risk of being delivered of a low birth weight infant at term. *Br J Obstet Gynaecol* 1978; 85:8.
44. Sokol RJ, Jone P, Chik L: Statistical enhancement of intrauterine growth retardation (IUGR) clinical risk detection. Scientific Program and Abstracts, 30th Annual Meeting of the Society for Gynecologic Investigation, Washington, DC, March 17-20, 1983.
45. Crane JP, Kopta MM: Prediction of intrauterine growth retardation via ultrasonically measured head/abdominal circumference ratios. *Obstet Gynecol* 1979; 54:597.
46. Neilson JP, Whitfield CR, Aitchison TC: Screening for the small-for-dates fetus: A two-stage ultrasonic examination schedule. *Br Med J* 1980; 280:1203.
47. Villar J, Belizan JM: The evaluation of the methods used in the diagnosis of intrauterine growth retardation. *Obstet Gynecol Surv* 1986; 41:187.

9

Evaluating the Diagnostic Use of Ultrasound and the Clinical Laboratory

José Villar, M.D., M.P.H., M.Sc.
José M. Belizán, M.D., Ph.D.

The need for early and adequate diagnosis of fetal growth retardation has been emphasized. However, to date there is no consensus on optimum timing for such a diagnostic test or whether the fetus will benefit most from intrauterine treatment or early delivery. If it is agreed that early and correct diagnosis of fetal growth retardation is a cornerstone of the obstetrician's approach to this syndrome, the method used should be carefully selected and only those techniques that provide the best results adopted. A long list of methods and techniques used for the diagnosis of intrauterine growth retardation (IUGR) has been proposed in the literature, and today many are used by obstetricians. However, they have seldom been evaluated using the correct epidemiologic methods or in the context of a screening program.

The methods used in the diagnosis of IUGR have been reviewed recently.[1–3] Reports of tests or laboratory techniques described as being highly successful in predicting IUGR appear frequently in the literature. The predictive value is frequently inflated because the studies are often performed in populations with very high incidence of IUGR. The higher the frequency of IUGR in the population, the more valuable the test will appear. However, the successful test results often disappear when the test is applied to the general obstetric population with a lower frequency of pregnancies with IUGR. Therefore in this chapter, in addition to presenting the results of methods suggested for IUGR diagnosis, we attempt to provide clinicians with a simple epidemiologic method to evaluate and select the clinical and laboratory techniques that can be incorporated or excluded from their obstetrical practice. Three recent excellent publications are recommended as additional reading on this topic.[4–6]

It is hoped that this will enable those devoted to patient care to utilize the literature and feel more confident with statistical or epidemiologic calculations that are often regarded as too complicated or mysterious.

METHOD OF ANALYSIS

One central issue is that in medicine it is always better to have an approximate answer to the correct question than the correct answer to an approximate question. Therefore we begin this chapter by presenting the main questions a clinician should consider before selecting a method for IUGR diagnosis. The terms "retrospective" and "prospective" used here are not related to the timing of data collection but to the chronologic position of the investigator vis-a-vis the test results when the question is formulated; that is, do we want to know what the test results were (retrospective) or how the test is able to predict pregnancy outcome (prospective).

Retrospective Evaluation

In the evaluation of a screening test, we can examine data from medical records and laboratory results and pose the following questions:

1. *Sensitivity*. What proportion of babies were correctly diagnosed as having IUGR during pregnancy by the method in question?
2. *Specificity*. What proportion of babies were correctly classified as having normal birth weight during pregnancy by the method in question?

The answers to these questions will help the obstetrician to decide: Is this a good method in itself independent of the population being examined?

After experimental results or those reported in the literature demonstrate that the method is good, the next question is: Will this technically good method be useful in my practice? This question is the most relevant for the clinician.

Prospective Evaluation

To evaluate performance of a screening test in a perinatal program or in obstetric practice, the following questions should be asked.

1. What is the probability that a patient with an abnormal test result

(e.g., abnormal sonogram) suggesting IUGR will actually deliver an infant with IUGR (positive predictive value, PPV)? Furthermore, what is the probability that this patient with an abnormal test result will have a baby with normal birth weight if labor is induced early (false positive)?

2. If the test result is normal (e.g., reactive nonstress test) and labor is not induced early, what is the probability that at term the baby will have IUGR (false negative)?

Knowing these probabilities will help the obstetrician integrate a test result with clinical judgment concerning the patient's characteristics and needs; the final clinical decision can then be made on the basis of all this information.

The main epidemiologic tool for calculating the probabilities listed above is the two-by-two table (Table 9–1). The rows in the table show the diagnostic status obtained from the test results (*fetal diagnosis*), for example nonreactive nonstress test or biparietal diameter (BPD) measurement below the 10th percentile. The columns show the true status obtained from the birth weight of the infant (*neonatal diagnosis*), classified as above or below a given cutoff point (e.g., 10th percentile) of a birth weight–gestational age distribution. Calculations that require only very simple arithmetic are presented at the bottom of the table. Table 9–2 exemplifies the directions of such calculations.

A given method with high sensitivity and PPV would lead to accurate prediction of IUGR and consequently promote timely and appropriate management of affected pregnancies. Conversely, a method with high false positive rates would yield a large number of normally growing fetuses receiving treatment for a nonexistent complication, with high costs and iatrogenic consequences. A high false negative rate implies that a large number of growth-retarded fetuses will not be detected and will be managed as normally growing fetuses.

It is important to note that these calculations are based on the separation of the population into two subgroups: IUGR and normal birth weight, using both test results and birth weight. When methods described in the literature are evaluated, the assumption is made that the cutoff points between normal and abnormal results selected for the clinical use of these methods are fixed and that they will always yield the best results. This may not be true; the evaluation of any of the methods should be originally performed at several possible cutoff points.

Furthermore, the definition of IUGR based on a given birth weight limit (e.g., ≤2500 gm) or percentile (e.g., 10th or lower) together with the population characteristics influence the incidence of IUGR in that population. These factors dramatically affect test performance. A discussion of these issues follows.

TABLE 9–1.
Data Layout and Formulas for Detecting IUGR*

Fetal Diagnosis		Neonatal Diagnosis (True Birth Weight Status) IUGR	Normal	Total
(Antepartum Diagnosed Status)	IUGR	a (Case detected)	b (False positive)	a + b
	Normal Fetal Growth	c (Case missed)	d (True normal)	c + d
	Total	a + c	b + d	N

Sensitivity = a/(a + c)
Specificity = d/(b + d)
False positive rate = b/(a + b)
False negative rate = c/(c + d)
True prevalence of IUGR = (a + c)/(a + b + c + d)
Positive predictive value (PPV) = a/(a + b)
Negative predictive value (NPV) = d/(c + d)
False positive rate = 1 − PPV
False negative rate = 1 − NPV
Positive predictive value (PPV) by prevalence level† =

$$\frac{\text{Sensitivity} \times \text{Prevalence}}{\text{Sensitivity} \times \text{Prevalence} + (1 - \text{Specificity})(1 - \text{Prevalence})}$$

*Adapted from Villar J, Belizán JM: *Obstet Gynecol Surv* 1986; 41:187.
†Data from Fleiss J: An introduction to applied probabilities, in *Statistical Methods for Rates and Proportion.* New York, John Wiley & Sons, pp 3–13; and Vecchio TJ: *N Engl J Med* 1966; 274:1171.

TABLE 9–2.
Rows and Columns Used in Calculations for the Evaluation of IUGR Diagnostic Tests*

		True Birth Weight Status IUGR	Normal		
Antepartum Diagnosed Status	IUGR	sensitivity	specificity	------→	Positive Predictive Value and False Positive
	Normal Fetal Growth			------→	False Negative
					Total

*Adapted from Stempel LE: *Am J Obstet Gynecol* 1982; 144:745; and Villar J, Belizán JM: *Obstet Gynecol Surv* 1986; 41:187.

DIAGNOSIS OF IUGR

From a review of 86 reports of methods for IUGR diagnosis published in English language journals between 1975 and 1983, 55 have information from which a two-by-two table may be constructed. Some of these reports discuss more than one test, in which case each test was considered independently. Definitions of abnormal intrauterine growth and outcome at birth (normal birth weight or IUGR) were accepted as the original authors have stated.

Methods reported are oriented to the identification of maternal risk factors, indirect or direct monitoring of fetal growth, measurement of metabolites produced totally or partially by the fetoplacental unit, or assessment of maternal metabolic functions.

Using the data layout and formulas[7,8] presented in Table 9–1, sensitivity and specificity of 42 methods were obtained and are plotted in Figure 9–1. An extensive description of the calculations and references can be obtained from Villar and Belizán.[1] As an example of these calculations, Table 9–3 presents data obtained from Odendaal et al.,[9] including calculations for sensitivity and specificity. The same calculations were performed for all methods shown in Figure 9–1. The diagonal line transecting the square refers to the level at which results are due to chance. The distance above the line up to the point of interest is inversely related to the predictability of the method. Parallel lines are drawn for a better estimation of this distance.

In Figure 9–1, for example, above the fourth parallel line there are 5 of 6 (83.3%) symbols for clinical methods, 16 of 20 (80%) for ultrasound measures, 5 of 8 (62.5%) for endocrine tests, and only 1 of 7 (14.3%) for antepartum cardiotocography. The highest value shown in the figure corresponds to three ultrasound measures: crown-rump length/trunk area[10] (sensitivity [Se] = 94.4%; specificity [Sp] = 87.9%); crown-rump length/trunk circumference[10] (Se = 88.9%; Sp = 91.1%); and amniotic fluid volume[11] (Se = 83.9%; Sp = 96.6%) (above the eighth parallel line in Figure 9–1). A clinical method, fundal height,[12] showed sensitivity 86.4% and specificity 89.5% (between the seventh and eighth parallel lines in Figure 9–1).

Another promising method not included in Figure 9–1 is the counting of fetal breathing movements, with sensitivity 60%, 71%, and 92.2% and specificity 85.9%, 91.8%, and 94.7% in three recent references.[13-15] Finally, fetal movements counting has been reported in one study,[16] with sensitivity 77% and specificity 86%.

Figure 9–2 summarizes PPV[7,8] (given in percent) calculated by using a standard incidence of IUGR of 10%. The best reported values for each technique from studies of a sample size of at least 100 cases are given. All values were calculated using the formula given in Table 9–1. For the example in Table 9–3, PPV is 16%, and false positive (1 - PPV) 84%. As can be seen in Figure 9–2, maternal risk factors and several clinical characteristics of the

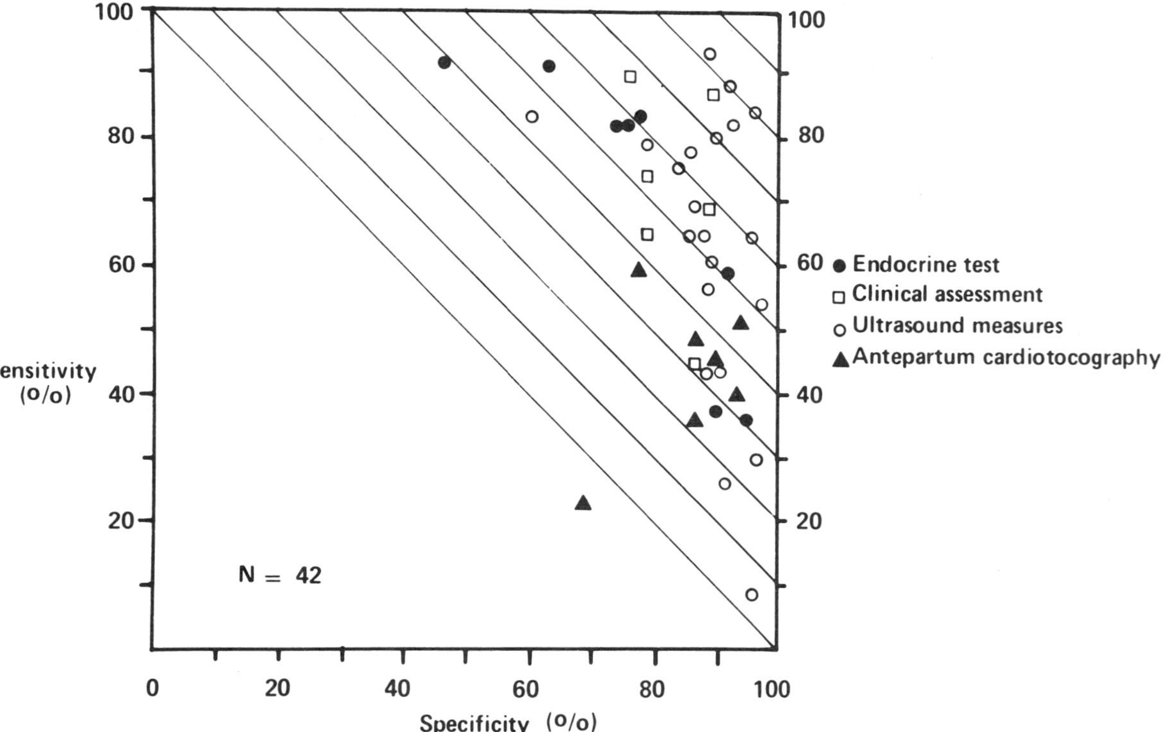

FIG 9–1.
Relationship between sensitivity and specificity of methods used in the diagnosis of intrauterine growth retardation (n = 42). Only reports with sample size greater than 100 and IUGR incidence above 1% to 2% are included. The closer to the central diagonal line the lower the predictability of the method. (Actual values from Villar J, Belizán JM: *Obstet Gynecol Surv* 1986; 41:187.)

TABLE 9–3.
Predictive Power of Placental Lactogen Hormone for the Diagnosis of IUGR*

		Neonatal Birthweight Status		
		IUGR	Normal	
Antepartum Diagnosed Status	IUGR	35	16	51
	Normal Fetal Growth	8	18	26
	Total	43	34	77

Sensitivity = a/(a + c)	35/43 = 81.4%
Specificity = d/(b + d)	18/34 = 52.9%
False positive = b/(a + b)	16/51 = 31.4%
False negative = c/(c + d)	8/26 = 30.8%
Positive predictive value = a/(a + b)	35/51 = 68.6%
Incidence of IUGR = (a + c)/(a + b + c + d)	43/77 = 55.8%
Positive predictive value† at IUGR incidence of 10%	† = 16%

*Data from Odendaal HJ, Malan C, Oosthuizen J: *S Afr Med J* 1981; 59:822.
†Formula given in Table 9–1 and references 7 and 8.

mother, including fundal height and weight gain by the thirty-fourth week of gestation, and the use of amniotic fluid volume or combinations of fetal ultrasound measurements are the procedures that can best identify IUGR.

Table 9–4 presents the median and range values for sensitivity and specificity (evaluation of the test in the laboratory) and false positive and false negative values (evaluation of the test in the obstetric practice for all groups of tests studied).

As can be appreciated, symphysis fundal height, hormones, and ultrasound methods rendered similar median values for sensitivity, while cardiotocography values are much lower. However, analyzing the ranges, BPD ultrasound measurements and hormones showed very low sensitivity values.

Hormones had a median value of 9.2% for false-negatives and very high upper range values (56.4%), implying that in some reports a large number of pregnancies with IUGR were not diagnosed by the method and were managed as normally-growing fetuses. All the studies with measurements of uterine fundal height and ultrasound showed false-negative rates below 13%.

EVALUATION OF METHODS FOR DETECTION OF IUGR AT DIFFERENT CUTOFF POINTS (IS THE TEST RESULT POSITIVE OR NEGATIVE?)

One question that is present during the development of a method for IUGR detection is: which is the best cutoff point of the test result for identifying

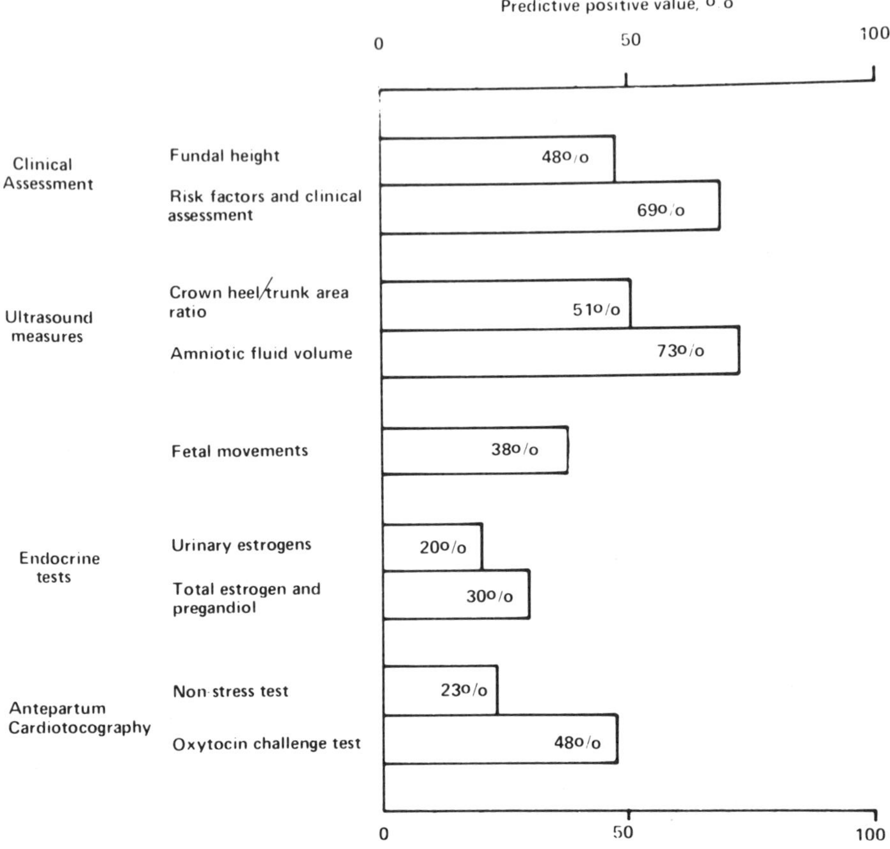

FIG 9–2.
Positive predictive value (PPV) at an IUGR incidence rate of 10% for selected methods used in the diagnosis of intrauterine growth retardation. Only the best reported value for each technique from studies of sample size of at least 100 were included. Crown-heel length/trunk area value represents average of three reports. (PPV calculated as suggested by Vecchio TJ: *N Engl J Med* 1966; 274:1171.)

IUGR fetuses? Tests used for IUGR detection have the possibility of using several cutoff points (e.g., risk factors, fetal movement count, urinary estrogens, ultrasound measurements). Moreover, when two different methods for IUGR detection are compared, this comparison should be conducted at several of the methods' cutoff points. This is necessary because it is possible that methods can be used in clinical situations at different cut-off points based on the objective pursued (actual diagnosis of IUGR versus screening). A very simple methodology can be implemented using the information presented in Table 9–1. For each cutoff point a two-by-two table is constructed and sensitivity and specificity are calculated. If a method is evaluated at three different cutoff points, three sets of specificity and sensitivity values should be obtained. If two methods are being compared, both should have the same information. These data are then plotted on a graph where the Y axis represents sensitivity and the X axis, one minus specificity. Each cutoff level for each method should contribute one point. The diagonal line does not represent a diagnostic value; an excellent test at all cutoff points will have the points close to the Y axis, with very few if any misclassifications.

This simplified approach for presenting and comparing two diagnostic tests at different cutoff levels, as well as for determining at which cutoff point a test offers the best predictive power for IUGR, is summarized in Table 9–5. This procedure only demonstrates the relationship between sensitivity and specificity and, therefore, is not affected by the incidence of IUGR. Clinicians and researchers are encouraged to use this tool. Other applications in obstetrics have been recently discussed by Richardson et al.[4] and Dierksheide.[17]

DETERMINING THE VALUE OF A TEST

To avoid the effect of IUGR incidence on the predictive value of the method, in Figure 9–2 PPV is recalculated assuming an IUGR incidence of 10% in all populations, using the formula given in Table 9–1. The PPV of a test increases directly with the incidence of the disease in the population, because a higher proportion of abnormal individuals in a population increases the probability that an abnormal test result will be present in the individual patient with IUGR.

We studied the relationship between PPV calculated for 66 different methods used in IUGR detection and the incidence of IUGR in the population in which those tests were applied (Fig 9–3). A positive and significant correlation was observed between these two variables ($R = 0.70$; $P < 0.01$). Therefore, independent of the test results, the higher the incidence of IUGR in the

TABLE 9–4.
Evaluation of Methods Used in the Diagnosis of IUGR*†

	Symphysis* fundal height	Hormones	Cardio-tocography (NST, OCT)	Combination of Ultrasound Measurements	Biparietal Diameter
Number of Reports	6	13	9	21	10
Sensitivity (%)	43.9–86.4	21.4–95	22–100	6.6–100	6.6–100
Median	66	71.4	48.4	69.4	60
Specificity (%)	79–89.5	45.3–94.6	67–94.1	60.3–100	84–97
Median	85	78.4	87	91.1	91
False Negative (%)	4.2–12.5	0.8–56.4	0–15.4	0–13	0–13
Median	6.3	9.2	8.2	4.9	5.6
False positive (%)	21–71	14–87	6.2–45.9	0–81.8	36–81.8
Median	56	50	27	55	56

†Ranges and medians are given for each group of studies.
*Data calculated from Villar J, Belizán JM: *Obstet Gynecol Surv* 1986; 41:187.

TABLE 9–5.
Evaluation of Screening Methods for IUGR Detection

1. Select the outcome variable as specific as possible in advance (definition of IUGR).
2. Select several logical cutoff points for the definition of abnormal test (abnormal fetal growth).
3. Construct a 2×2 table for each cutoff point of interest. Calculate sensitivity and specificity for each one.
4. Plot in a graph for each cutoff point sensitivity (y) and 1-specificity (x). Select the best cutoff point for your test or select the best test at a given cutoff point if comparison between tests is the objective.
5. Calculate the incidence of IUGR in the studied population.
6. Calculate the positive predictive value and the false-positive rate for that population.
7. Using the formula in Table 1, calculate the positive predictive value for a range of IUGR incidences. Use this information in your recommendations for the use of the test in other populations.

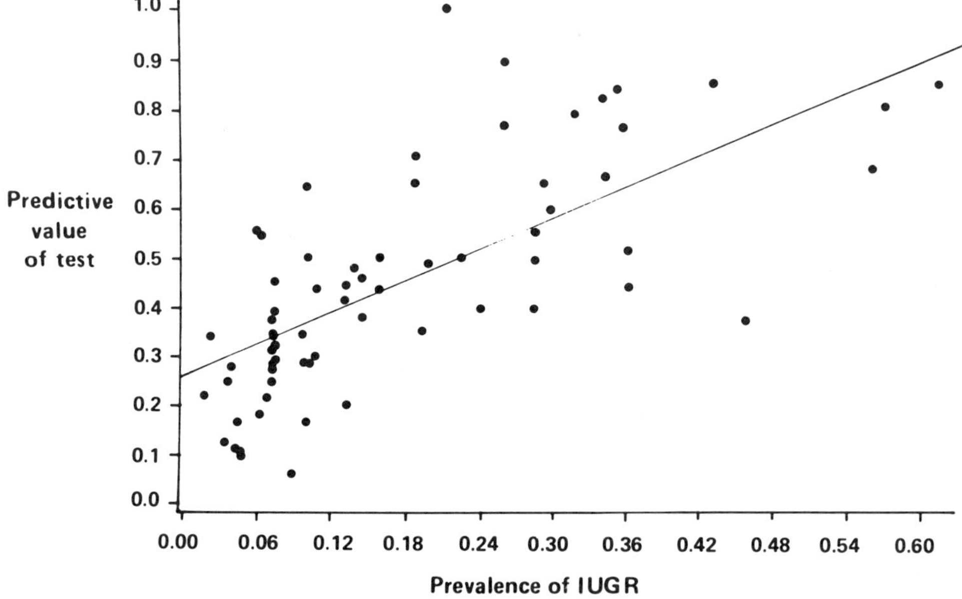

FIG 9–3.
Relationship between IUGR prevalence and the predictive value of the test. Sixty-six different procedures were included. The higher the IUGR incidence the better the predictability of the method ($R = 0.70$, $\beta = 1.08$, $P < 0.001$). (Adapted from Villar J, Belizán JM: *Obstet Gynecol Surv* 1986; 41:187.)

population the higher the PPV. It is relevant to observe a high correlation in spite of the use of completely different methods, operations, and populations. Controlling for sensitivity and specificity, a regression model of the PPV-IUGR prevalence relationship showed the same linear relationship at two levels of sensitivity. Therefore, regardless of the sensitivity or specificity of the procedure, the prevalence of IUGR in the population under consideration explains about 50% (r^2 = 49%) of the PPV variability.

As an example, let us consider a study evaluating the use of human placental lactogen to predict IUGR.[9] The authors reported sensitivity 81.4%, specificity 52.9%, and PPV 68.6%, with an IUGR incidence of 55.8% (43 of 77). It is clear that this population is a high-risk group, with more than half of all of the pregnancies delivering an infant with IUGR. Suppose now that we would like to use this method in a general population where it can be estimated that the incidence of IUGR is 10%. Using the PPV formula provided in Table 9–1, PPV 68.6% for a population with incidence of IUGR 55.8% decreases to 16% in a population with 10% incidence of babies with IUGR. This population with 10% IUGR incidence is the most likely encountered by the obstetrician.

DISCUSSION

In the analysis of the PPV of a test, the incidence of IUGR in the population must be taken into account. Frequently, a new method is developed in a the reports focused only on the diagnosis of IUGR (sensitivity), and no information is given on the diagnosis of normally grown fetuses (specificity). Changing the cutoff point of the method could substantially improve sensitivity, but will always imply a decrease in specificity. In this case the method will not only diagnose a higher percentage of IUGR but in addition would diagnose IUGR in a larger number of fetuses with normal intrauterine growth. This would imply that a higher number of normal pregnancies will require special care, increasing cost and sometimes the possibility of iatrogenic complications.

It should be remembered that the selection of the final cutoff point should not be based only on the laboratory results. Factors to be considered include the probability of fetal death if IUGR is not detected, the treatments available for use by the obstetrician, the cost and risks of the treatments, and the side effects of these treatments when applied to healthy pregnancies misclassified as IUGR. All of these considerations should be considered before incorporating a new test into clinical practice.

In the analysis of the PPV of a test, the incidence of IUGR in the population must be taken into account. Frequently, a new method is developed in a population with a high incidence of IUGR (such as in a tertiary center or university hospital). Later, when it is used in a low-risk population with a lower incidence of IUGR, the reported results will be less promising. Figure 9–3 and the formula in Table 9–1 provide tools to calculate the expected PPV in one specific population. This analysis should always be performed before introduction of a new test or replacement of an old method (see Table 9–5).

It is evident that when combining maternal risk factors with clinical indices (e.g., fundal height, weight gain monitoring), as in Wennergren and Karlsson,[18] excellent IUGR predictability is obtained. To obtain these results, certain conditions not often found in clinical practice must be considered. Clinicians usually collect a large amount of information, including previous obstetric history, but seldom make good use of it.[19] Furthermore, clinical measurements that require graphic plotting at each prenatal visit, such as fundal height and maternal weight gain, to allow better interpretation of the results, seldom are used.

It is also evident from the data that the measurement of BPD by ultrasound is not a better screening technique than are other clinical measurements such as fundal height. The recent report from the National Institutes of Health[20] on ultrasound supports this interpretation. On the contrary, the use of the ratio of two morphometric measurements using ultrasound imaging[10] gives an excellent prediction rate of IUGR. These reports, however, included an early (15 weeks) BPD measurement for accurate assessment of gestational age. This policy requires early contact with patients plus routine BPD measurement in all patients, which is not recommended at this time.[20] Qualitative amniotic fluid volume determination[11] and sonographically detected oligohydramnios[21] appear to be complementary techniques. However, these data should be reproduced in larger studies and the methods standardized before its universal recommendation.

In short, a combination of morphometric measurements with the evaluation of amniotic fluid volume represents the best ultrasound alternative for IUGR detection. The need for accurate dating, the use of real-time ultrasound (not always available), the cost, and to some extent the concern about safety limit the utility of these techniques for routine screening and reserve them for specific medical indications.[20]

Fetal cardiotocography (nonstress test, oxytocin challenge test) and hormonal values do not contribute to a better rate of prediction of IUGR when the above methods are applied. Fetal movement counting has been suggested as an attractive method for monitoring fetal well-being. Based on information in malnourished children, reduction in activity could be expected as an adaptive mechanism in fetuses with IUGR. Preliminary data on the capacity of this technique to predict IUGR are encouraging, and fetal movement counting in a randomized controlled trial showed a statistically significant lower stillbirth rate than in a group followed with routine procedures.[22] Its simplicity and low cost make fetal movement counting attractive for first-level care, yet its noncompliance rate of 22% also suggests that its use may be limited to a well-motivated population.[22]

In diagnosis of IUGR, we recommend thorough evaluation of the maternal history, with careful follow-up of fundal height measurements and maternal weight increase, plotting the values on standard charts. Pregnancies suspected by these methods or by clinical or obstetric history of being IUGR should be reevaluated by ultrasound by using a combination of morphometric measurements and evaluation of amniotic fluid volume.

Previous methods for diagnosing IUGR[23,24] are constantly replaced by new laboratory and ultrasound techniques.[25,26] In order to assist in determining which of the newer diagnostic methods are accurate, readers are strongly encouraged to adopt our simple method of evaluation, apply it to the data at hand, and reach their own conclusions. It is only in this practical way that clinicians will be confident enough to utilize statistical techniques and will not be used by them.

REFERENCES

1. Villar J, Belizán JM: The evaluation of the methods used in the diagnosis of intrauterine growth retardation. *Obstet Gynecol Surv* 1986; 41:187.
2. Neilson JP, Munjanja SP, Mooney R, et al: Product of fetal crown-rump length and trunk area: Ultrasound measurement of high-risk pregnancies. *Br J Obstet Gynaecol* 1984; 91:756.
3. Department of Obstetrics, St. George's Hospital Medical School, London. An end to antenatal oestrogen monitoring? *Lancet* 1984; 1:1171.
4. Richardson D, Schwartz S, Weinbaum P, et al: Diagnostic tests in obstetrics: A method for improved evaluation. *Am J Obstet Gynecol* 1985; 152:613.
5. Stempel LE: Eenie, meenie, minie, mo . . . what do the data really show? *Am J Obstet Gynecol* 1982; 144:745.
6. Grant A, Mohide P: Screening and diagnostic tests in antenatal care, in *Effectiveness and Satisfaction in Antenatal Care*, Clinics in Developmental Medicine, No 81/82, 1982, p 22.
7. Fleiss J: An introduction to applied probabilities, in *Statistical Methods for Rates and Proportion*. New York, John Wiley & Sons, 1981, pp 3–13.
8. Vecchio TJ: Predictive value of a single diagnostic test in unselected populations. *N Engl J Med* 1966; 274:1171.
9. Odendaal HJ, Malan C, Oosthuizen J: Hormonal placental functions and intrauterine growth retardation in patients with positive contraction stress test. *S Afr Med J* 1981; 59:822.
10. Neilson JP, Whitfield CR, Aitchison TC: Screening for the small-for-dates fetus: A two-stage ultrasonic examination schedule. *Br Med J* 1980; 281:247.
11. Manning FA, Hill LM, Platt LD: Qualitative amniotic fluid volume determination by ultrasound: Antepartum detection of intrauterine growth retardation. *Am J Obstet Gynecol* 1981; 139:255.
12. Belizán JM, Villar J, Nardin JC, et al: Diagnosis of intrauterine growth retardation by a simple clinical method: Measurement of uterine height. *Am J Obstet Gynecol* 1978; 131:643.
13. Manning FA, Platt LD, Sipos L, et al: Fetal breathing movements and the nonstress test in high-risk pregnancies. *Am J Obstet Gynecol* 1979; 135:511.
14. Platt LD, Manning FA, Lemay M, et al: Human fetal breathing: Relationship to fetal condition. *Am J Obstet Gynecol* 1978; 132:514.
15. Manning FA: Fetal breathing movements as a reflection of fetal status. *Postgrad Med* 1977; 61:116.

16. Jarvis GJ, MacDonald HN: Fetal movement in small-for-dates babies. *Br J Obstet Gynaecol* 1979; 86:724.
17. Dierksheide WC: Receiver operating characteristic analysis of glycosylated hemoglobin and the standard test for carbohydrate intolerance in pregnancy. *Am J Obstet Gynecol* 1985; 153:113.
18. Wennergren M, Karlsson K: A scoring system for antenatal identification of fetal growth retardation. *Br J Obstet Gynaecol* 1982; 89:520.
19. Chng PK, Hall MH, MacGillivray I: An audit of antenatal care: The value of the first antenatal visit. *Br Med J* 1980; 281:1184.
20. NICHD-FDA. *Diagnostic Ultrasound Imaging in Pregnancy*. Bethesda, Md, US Department of Health and Human Services, NIH Publication No 84-667, 1984.
21. Sokol RJ, Philipson EH, Williams T: Clinical detection of intrauterine growth retardation improved by sonographically diagnosed oligohydramnios. Presented at the Annual Meeting of the Society for Gynecology Investigation, Washington, DC, March 1983.
22. Neldan S: Fetal movements as an indicator of fetal well being. *Lancet* 1980; 1:1222.
23. Wolfrum R, Bordasch C, Holweg J, et al: Prognostic value of combined assay of total estrogen and pregnanediol in 24 hour urine: Experience with 500 pregnancies in an endocrine surveillance program during the second trimester. *J Perinat Med* 1977; 5:10.
24. Hayden BL, Simpson JL, Ewing DE, et al: Can the oxytocin challenge test serve as the primary method for managing high-risk pregnancies? *Obstet Gynecol* 1975; 46:251.
25. Brown HL, Miller JM, Gabert HA: Ultrasonic recognition of the small-for-gestational age fetus. *Obstet Gynecol* 1987; 69:631.
26. Haddow JE, Palomaki GE, Knight GJ: Can low birth weight after elevated maternal serum alpha-fetoprotein be explained by maternal weight? *Obstet Gynecol* 1987; 70:26.

10

Ultrasonic Measurements for Diagnosis

Peter A. T. Grannum, M.D.

The traditional method used by the obstetrician to assess fetal growth has been measurement of fundal height and monitoring of maternal weight gain. Both observations are notoriously poor for diagnosing intrauterine growth retardation (IUGR) and for following fetal growth. A recent study examining the accuracy of fundal growth in determining IUGR resulted in sensitivity 64% and positive predictive value 29%.[1] These two values should be used only as a screening tool. Patients with risk factors (see Chapters 5 and 8) with or without lagging fundal growth or adequate weight gain should be observed with ultrasonic measurements to follow fetal growth and to diagnose IUGR. Although ultrasonic measurements do not guarantee 100% accuracy in the diagnosis of IUGR, the sensitivity and positive predictive value can be significantly improved.

On ultrasonography the fetus can be viewed as having two major components: head and body. Measurements used to reflect head growth include biparietal diameter and head circumference; abdominal circumference is used to follow growth of the body. In symmetric growth retardation both components fall off the growth curve established for the particular fetus. This is referred to as type I, or concordant, growth retardation. If there is normal head growth but the body falls off the growth curve, asymmetric growth is diagnosed (discordant, or type II). These two abnormal growth patterns are closely linked to the timing of the in utero insult. If the insult occurs early (i.e., before 20 weeks, the time of maximum skeletal growth and cell hyperplasia), both fetal length and weight will be affected (type I).[2] If the insult occurs after 20 weeks, the major effects will be less subcutaneous tissue and decreased glycogen stores in the fetal liver, resulting in low fetal weight (type II). Insults that lead to symmetric growth retardation include first-trimester fetal exposure to drugs and viral agents (see Chapter 5). Chromosomal aberrations (e.g., trisomies 13 and 18) also affect growth. Poor nutrition, smoking, and toxemia of pregnancy are more likely to affect the fetus in the second and third trimesters, and result in an asymmetric growth pattern. The fetus with asymmetric IUGR allowed to remain in a hostile uterine environment may eventually become symmetrically growth retarded.

DIAGNOSIS

The diagnosis of normal or abnormal fetal growth depends on the assessment of fetal age and fetal weight. When dates are known or have been confirmed by ultrasound examination in the first trimester or first half of the second trimester, the diagnosis of abnormal growth can be more securely recognized. If the dates are unknown and IUGR is suspected, the diagnosis is more difficult because the parameters used to assess age and weight may also be affected. In addition to age and weight measurements, other parameters such as the intrauterine environment and the qualitative assessment of fetal age and maturity (placental grading, amniotic fluid, and ossification centers) may assist in the diagnosis and antepartum management. Charts of the various ultrasound measures of fetal growth are presented in Appendixes 10–1 to 10–8.

FETAL AGE

The diagnosis of IUGR is heavily dependent on fetal age. In the first half of pregnancy there is less variation in fetal size than in the second half. Crown-rump measurement in the first trimester is accurate within ± 4.7 days.[3,4] In patients at high risk for a fetus with IUGR (Chapters 5 and 8) dating should be performed early in the pregnancy. Knowledge of the true gestational age of a fetus suspected of having IUGR will enhance diagnostic accuracy.

The following measurements can be used to determine gestational age once IUGR is suspected.

Biparietal Diameter

Fetal biparietal diameter (BPD) is commonly used to estimate age of the fetus. It is technically one of the easiest measurements to obtain. If BPD is used alone to diagnose abnormal growth or to follow fetal growth, only 44% to 75% of growth-retarded fetuses are detected.[5,6] The most likely reason for this rests in the differentiation of symmetric and asymmetric growth patterns.

In asymmetric IUGR (type II), BPD will continue to grow appropriately or close to it, whereas the body values will fall off the growth curve; hence this form of IUGR will be missed. In symmetric IUGR (type I, or concordant), the BPD value falls off the growth curve along with the body value. A lag in growth of the BPD is considered only when it is noted for more than 2 weeks.

To obtain BPD, measurements are taken at right angles to the fetal spine, over the parietal eminences of the calvarium (Fig 10–1). Flexion and extension of the fetal head and posterior and anterior asynclitism necessitate manipulation of the transducer to obtain the necessary anatomic landmarks. The anatomic landmarks needed to ensure the correct scanning plane include the midline, thalami, septum pellucidum, and insula (sylvian fissure area with pulsating middle cerebral artery). The maximum diameter is obtained, and the measurements are taken from leading edge to leading edge (Fig 10–2).

Errors in measurement of BPD (and other fetal values) include lack of attention to anatomic landmarks, poor technique, and faulty machine calibration. In addition, overestimation and underestimation of BPD can be related to changes in shape of the fetal head.

Cephalic Index

Although cephalic index cannot be used to estimate fetal age, changes in shape of the fetal head may lead to underestimation or overestimation of BPD. Dolichocephaly, or flattening of the fetal head, is often seen in premature rupture of the membranes, in the premature fetus, and in breech presentation. Brachycephaly ("round head") leads to overestimation of BPD. Fetal age, fetal weight, and head-to-body ratio depend on accurate determination of BPD; thus Hadlock et al.[7] proposed using cephalic index to determine whether BPD can be used in these estimations.[7]

The cephalic index is obtained by measuring BPD and occipitofrontal diameter (OFD) using the same anatomic landmarks as for BPD. The OFD is measured between the outer margins of the calvarium, perpendicular to the BPD (Fig 10–3). Cephalic index is expressed as

$$CI = \frac{OFD}{BPD} \times 100$$

If cephalic index is between 75% and 85%, BPD can be used for dating or estimating fetal weight. Outside this range other values should be used.

Head Circumference

Using the same anatomic landmarks as for BPD, head circumference can be calculated by measuring the two diameters of the fetal head (BPD and

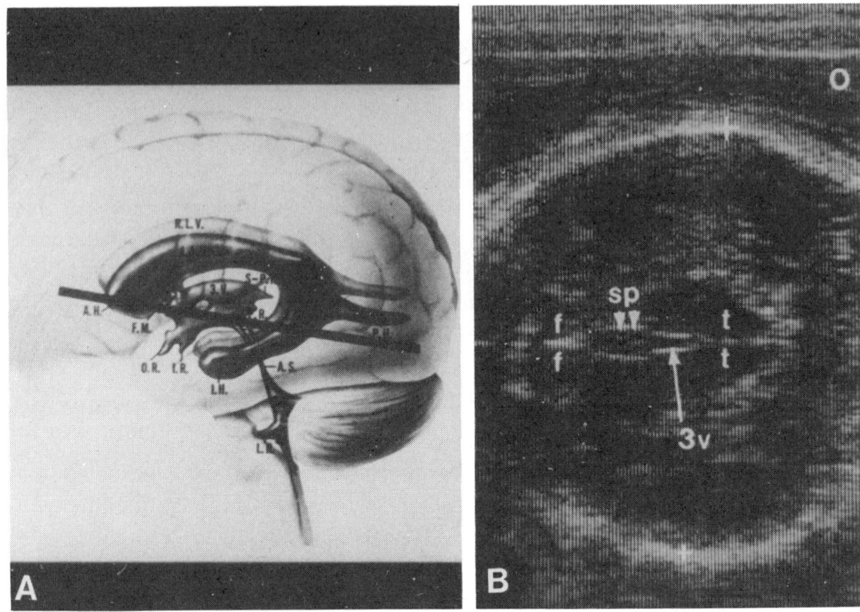

FIG 10–1.
A, drawing of fetal brain showing scan plane for biparietal diameter. **B,** scan highlighting anatomic landmarks for biparietal diameter.

OFD) taken perpendicular to each other (Fig 10–4).[8] The circumference can be calculated from the formula

$$\frac{D_1 + D_2}{2} \times \pi$$

Orbital Measurements

Outer and inner orbital measurements can be used for dating.[9] Measurements for the outer orbital distances are taken from the outer margins of the orbits; the inner orbital measurement is the distance from the medial borders of both orbits (Fig 10–5). Hypotelorism and hypertelorism, which may be associated with congenital malformations, preclude the use of these measurements for dating.

Long Bone Measurements

Measurements of the femur and other long bones such as the humerus, ulna, and tibia can be used for dating.[10–12] The bone length measurements vary, as do all fetal parameters, according to genetic disposition, malnutrition, and type and timing of the in utero insult. With severe IUGR femur length may be shorter than expected. The femur is the easiest bone to measure.

If the spine is followed to the sacral area longitudinally and the transducer is rotated ventrally from the spine using the sacral tip as the rotating point, a longitudinal view of the femoral bone is obtained (Fig 10–6). The measurements should be taken from the area just medial to the greater trochanteric process to the distal femoral end.

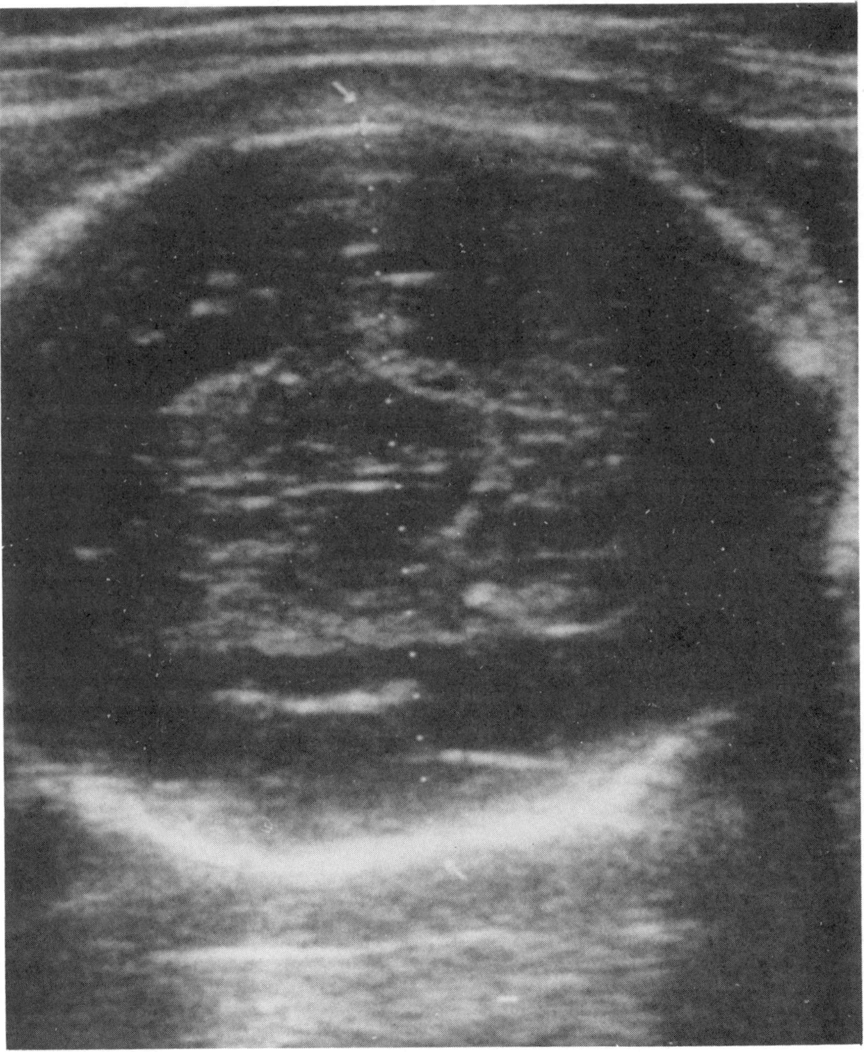

FIG 10–2.
Biparietal diameter. Note calipers are placed at leading edge to leading edge (*arrows*).

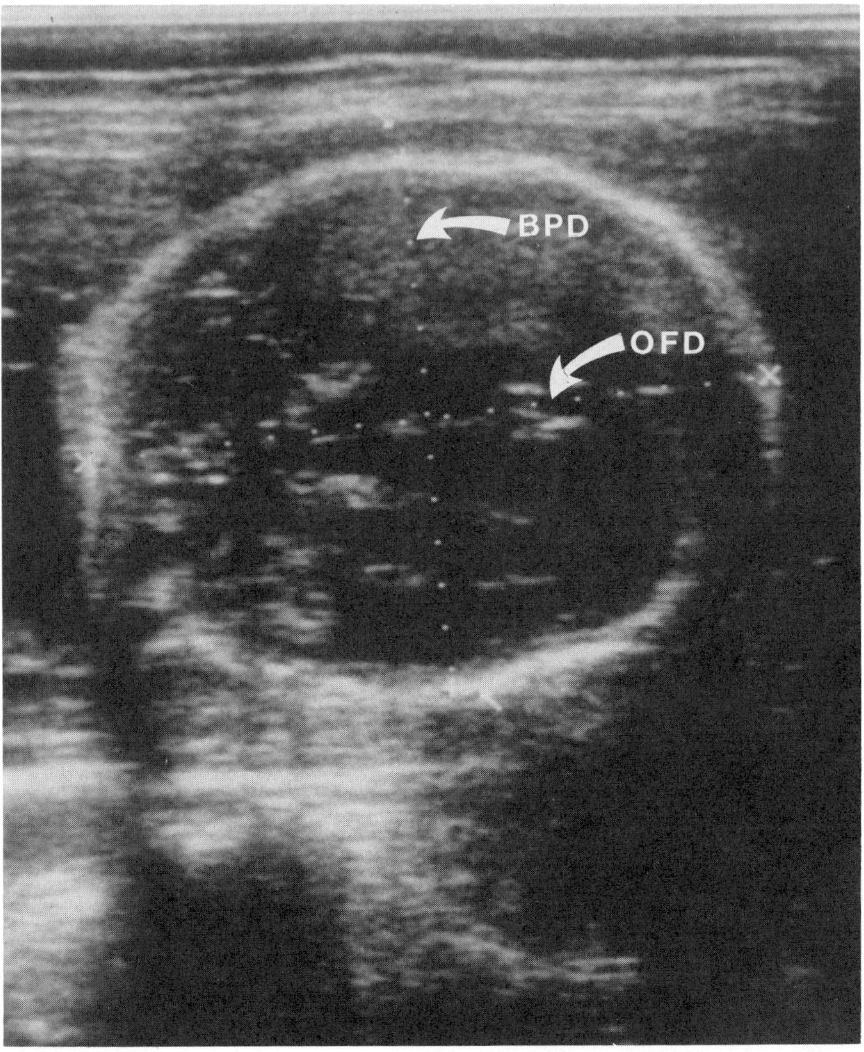

FIG 10–3.
Cephalic index. Occipitofrontal diameter (OFD) is measured between the outer margins of the calvarium, perpendicular to the biparietal diameter (BPD).

Abdominal Circumference

Abdominal circumference is not an accurate parameter for estimating gestational age.[13] It is far more useful for distinguishing the two types of growth patterns and for estimation of fetal weight. In experiments with chronically nutritionally deprived animals, the liver was the most severely affected organ.[14] Glycogen stores were rapidly depleted. Inasmuch as the liver accounts for most of the upper abdominal girth, measurements of abdominal circumference should be taken in the upper abdomen.

A transverse section of the fetal abdomen is taken at the level of the umbilical vein as the left hepatic vein meets the right hepatic vein (Fig 10–7,A). The two diameters of the fetal abdomen are obtained perpendicular to each other and between the outer edges of the abdominal contour (see Fig 10–7,A). The circumference is calculated from the formula

$$\text{Circumference} = \frac{D_1 + D_2}{2} \times \pi$$

Abdominal circumference should not be measured at the level where the umbilical vein meets the maternal abdominal wall (Fig 10–7,B). When the fetus is in the prone position, the umbilical vein will not be visible. In this view the landmarks should include the fetal kidneys and stomach (Fig 10–8).

An alternative method of determining the circumference is to trace the abdominal contour using the calipers on the ultrasound machine (see Fig 10–8). This may be more accurate when the fetal abdomen appears elliptical, as frequently seen when there is severe oligohydramnios and the abdomen is compressed by a fetal limb.

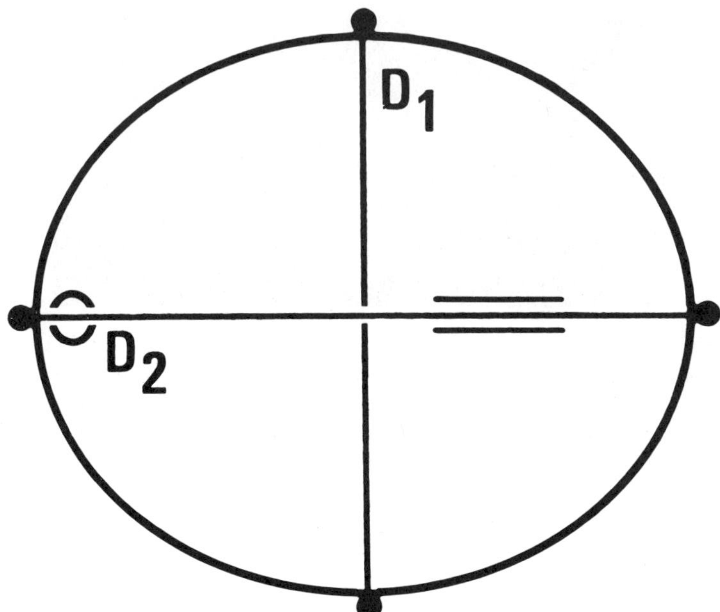

FIG 10–4.
Both head circumference and abdominal circumference are measured between their outer margins.

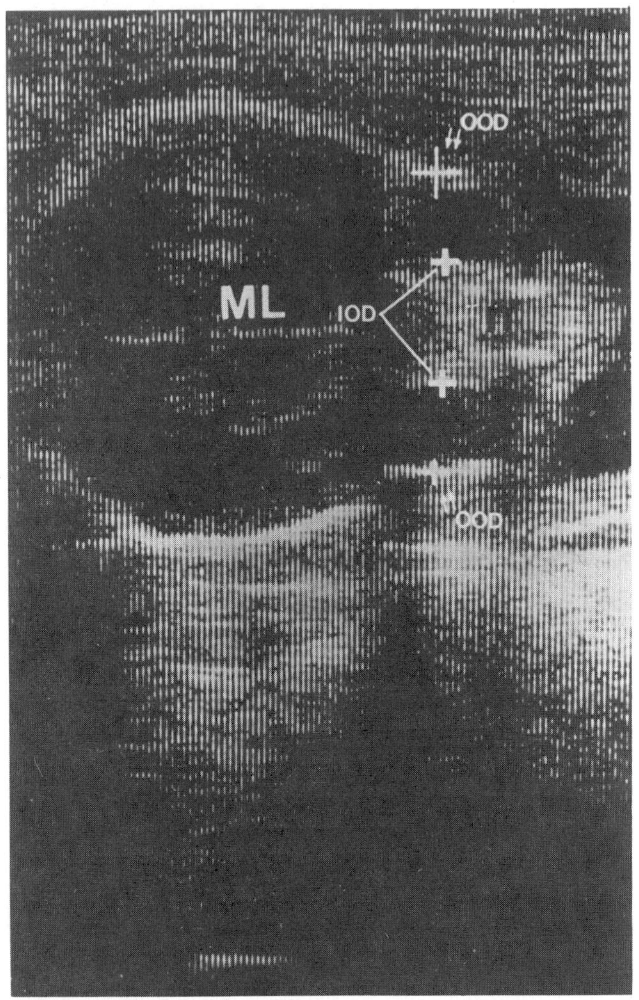

FIG 10–5.
Orbital measurements. The inner orbital diameter (IOD) is the distance from the medial borders of both orbits; the outer orbital diameter is measured from the outer margins of the orbits. *ML* = midline. (From Mayden KL, et al: Orbital diameters: A new parameter for prenatal diagnosis and dating. *Am J Obstet Gynecol* 1982; 144:289. Used by permission.)

ESTIMATED FETAL WEIGHT

Fetal weight can be estimated by BPD and abdominal circumference. The formula of Shepard et al.[15] (modified from Warsof's original formula) should be used. The standard error has been calculated to be approximately 10% in the small or average-size fetus. The BPD should be rechecked with the cephalic index to avoid overestimation or underestimation, which would directly affect fetal weight estimation.

If the BPD is unavailable or the cephalic index indicates it should not be used, the femur length and abdominal circumference can be combined to estimate fetal weight.[16]

The calculated in utero weight can be compared with the ultrasonographic fetal weight/gestational age curves such as those derived by Ott and Doyle.[17] These authors found 90% sensitivity and 80% specificity in the detection of IUGR when estimated fetal weight was compared with the normal curve. Some centers use the Lubchenco et al.[18] original birth weight curves for comparison.

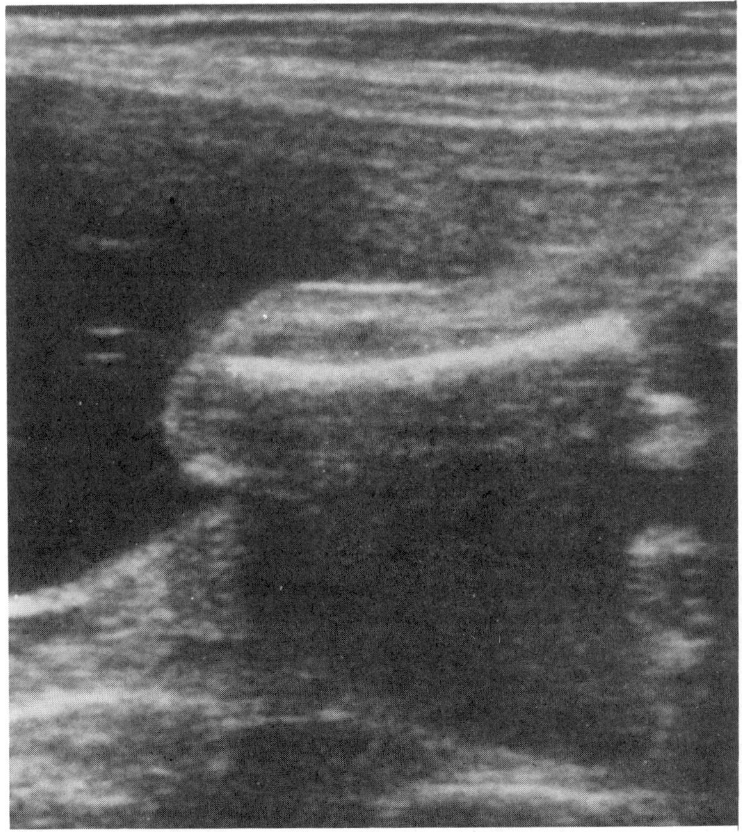

FIG 10–6.
Femur length measurement. Calipers are placed from the area just medial to the greater trochanteric process to the distal femoral end.

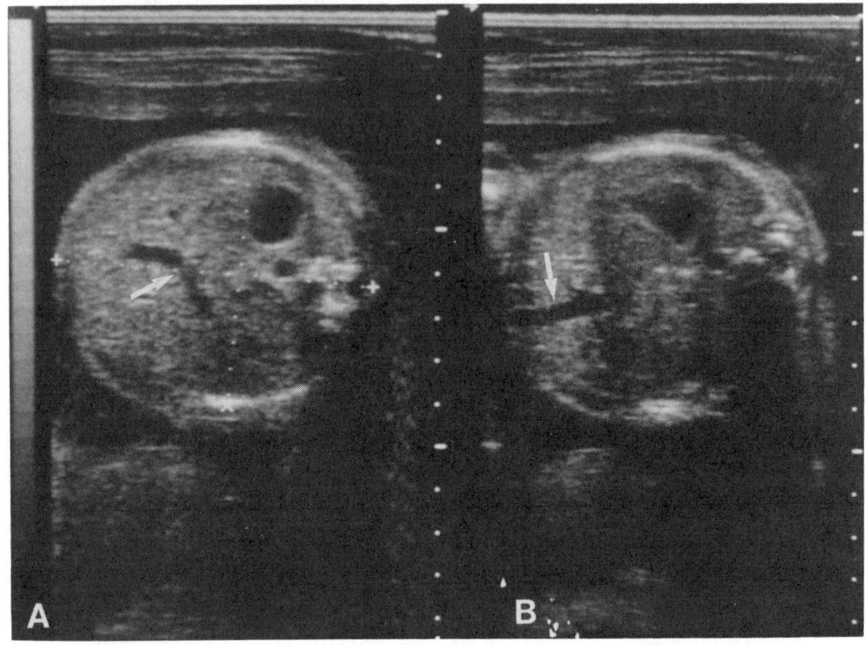

FIG 10–7.
A, abdominal circumference taken at the level of the left hepatic vein where it meets the right hepatic vein. **B,** incorrect level for measuring abdominal circumference. Here the umbilical vein is at the maternal abdominal wall.

HEAD-TO-BODY RATIO (HEAD CIRCUMFERENCE TO ABDOMINAL CIRCUMFERENCE RATIO)

In general, head circumference exceeds abdominal circumference until approximately 32 weeks. After 32 weeks, due to the significant deposition of fat and subcutaneous tissue, the ratio declines, dropping below unity after 36 weeks gestation.[19] The head-to-body ratio is used to differentiate the asymmetric and symmetric forms of IUGR. If the ratio is above the 95th percentile and estimated fetal weight is below the 10th percentile, the fetus is considered to have asymmetric growth retardation; if the estimated fetal weight is below the 10th percentile and the head-to-body ratio is normal, symmetric growth retardation should be suspected.

Crane and Kopta[20] prospectively studied 47 patients at risk for IUGR. Thirty-seven fetuses had a normal head-to-body ratio, and all were appropriate for gestational age at birth; ten fetuses had elevated ratios, and all were growth retarded.

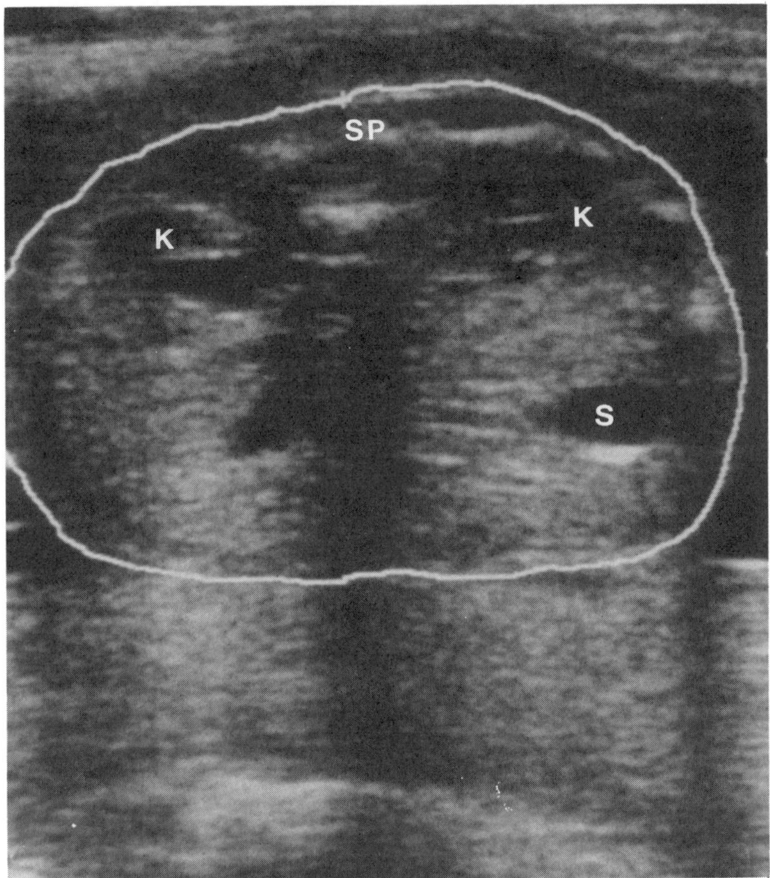

FIG 10–8.
Abdominal circumference in the fetus in the prone position. Landmarks are the fetal kidneys (*K*), stomach (*S*), and spine (*Sp*).

EPIPHYSEAL ASSESSMENT

The distal femoral epiphysis and proximal tibial epiphysis are usually detectable by 32 and 36 weeks, respectively.[21] The calcaneal ossification center can be identified at 24 weeks and the tarsal ossification center by 26 weeks[21] in the fetus with symmetric IUGR. Gentili et al.[22] found the distal femoral epiphysis to be absent in 41% of cases, small in 25%, and normal in 33.3%. Epiphyseal assessment cannot be used to date a pregnancy. When dates are unknown, presence or absence of the ossification centers may be useful in antepartum management and in assigning gestational age.

AMNIOTIC FLUID VOLUME

Quantification of amniotic fluid volume has remained a problem for the sonographer and sonologist. There is no method clinically applicable for determining amniotic fluid volume. Scanning the small parts of the fetus allows the best view for the assessment of fluid. If there is space between the fetal elbows and the knees, ample fluid can be said to be present. It is important to realize that the quantity of amniotic fluid normally decreases in the third trimester. Knowledge of the approximate amounts of fluid at different periods of gestation comes from experience. A frequent finding in IUGR is oligohydramnios. The cause is proposed to be decreased fetal renal blood flow with subsequent low urine output.

Manning et al.[23] examined 120 patients with a diagnosis of IUGR. Low fluid volume was diagnosed if the pockets of fluid measured less than 1 cm. Of 29 patients with low amniotic fluid volume, 26 delivered growth-retarded fetuses. Oligohydramnios with IUGR should prompt a search for other congenital abnormalities, especially when noted before 20 weeks gestation (or 24 to 26 weeks in most centers). Amniocentesis should be offered, and the fluid should be sent for culture for TORCH infections and chromosomal studies. Mercer et al.[24] reported a 7% malformation rate in patients with oligohydramnios without ruptured membranes.

PLACENTAL GRADING

As pregnancy advances, the placenta changes in configuration. Four grades were described by Grannum et al.[25] (Fig 10–9). Three areas of the placenta were highlighted: the chorionic plate, the placental substance, and the basal layer area. All placentas start as grade 0. The chorionic plate is smooth; the substance and basal layer areas are devoid of echogenic densities. In the grade I placenta the chorionic plate is more indented and the substance has linear echogenic densities; the basal layer area is devoid of densities. In the grade II placenta, in addition to the linear echogenic densities in the placental substance, the basal layer demonstrates echogenic densities. These are linear and are parallel to the long axis of the placenta. The linear densities (intercotyledonary septa) between the chorionic plate and the basal layer are incomplete. In the grade III placenta the linear densities extend from the chorionic plate to the basal layer area without a break.

The mean time of development from grade 0 to I is 31.1 weeks; from grade I to II, 36.6 weeks; and from grade II to III, 38.8 weeks.[26] Kazzi et al.[27] studied 109 pregnancies in which fetal birth weight was less than 2,700 gm. A grade III placenta was associated with infants small for gestational age 59% of the time, and grade I and II placentas 25% of the time (sensitivity 62%, specificity 73%, predictive value 59%). Although this test may be inappropriate

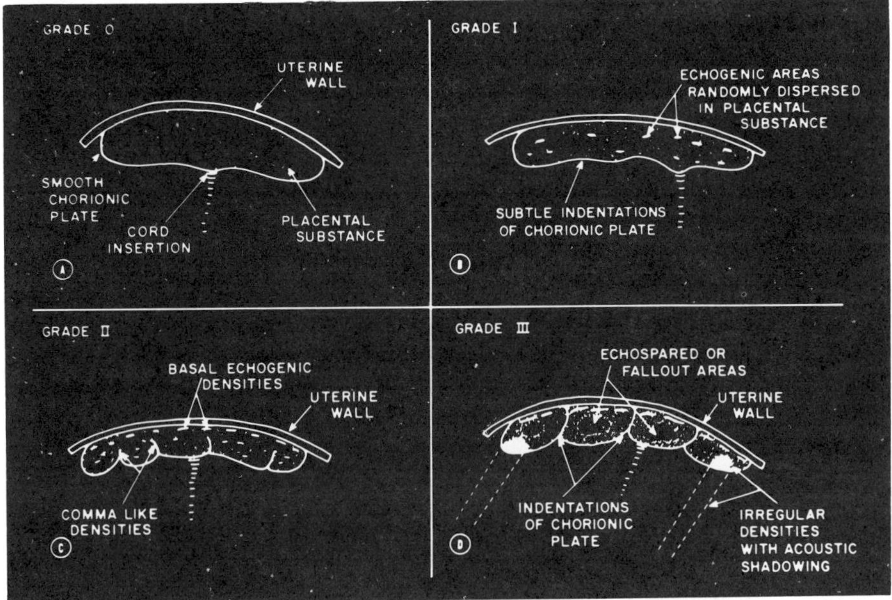

FIG 10–9.
Diagram of placental grades 0 through III. (From Grannum PAT, et al: The ultrasonic changes in the maturing placenta and their relation to fetal pulmonic maturity. *Am J Obstet Gynecol* 1979; 133:915. Used by permission.)

for diagnosing IUGR, it is a useful adjunct to other tests because it offers information about the intrauterine environment, especially when dating is uncertain.

INTERPRETATION OF RESULTS

Guidelines for interpretation of ultrasound results for diagnosis of IUGR are given in Table 10–1.

Recently, Doppler ultrasound has been applied to the analysis of the blood flow of the fetoplacental unit and uterine arteries (see Chapter 11). Griffin et al.[28] measured pulsatility index from the waveforms of the uterine or arcuate arteries in normal and IUGR pregnancies. The pulsatility index is a measure of resistance. In normal pregnancies there is a decline in pulsatility index in the second trimester, with a concomitant increase in diastolic frequency. Patients with IUGR had decreased diastolic frequencies and elevated pulsatility indices. The increased resistance may be related to the failure of trophoblastic invasion of the spiral arteries, which occurs in the second trimester.[29,30] Failure of invasion is seen in pregnancies complicated by preeclampsia and IUGR. Studies are under way to determine whether IUGR can be predicted from the evaluation of the waveforms of the umbilical artery.[31,32] In addition, the technology is now available to study blood flow in the uterine artery.[33] Further studies are needed to assess the application of this method in the diagnosis and management of IUGR.

CONCLUSION

The accuracy of the diagnosis of IUGR can be enhanced if the physician exercises careful and consistent attention to the patient's risk factors and the clinical landmarks such as fundal height assessment and maternal weight

TABLE 10–1.
Interpretation of Ultrasound Results for the Diagnosis of IUGR

Parameter*	Results	Diagnosis	Disposition
BPD	Appropriate for dates (within 2 weeks of dates)	No IUGR	Repeat only if clinical parameters warrant.
EFW	Above 10th birth weight percentile		
H/A ratio	In normal range		
Amniotic fluid volume	Normal		
BPD	Appropriate for dates (within 2 weeks of dates)	Probable asymmetric IUGR	Repeat ultrasound examination every 2 weeks if not delivered.
EFW	Below 10th birth weight percentile		Start antepartum surveillance and continue until delivery
H/A ratio	Above 95th percentile		
Amniotic fluid volume	Low		
BPD	Two weeks or more Smaller than expected for menstrual dates	Probable symmetric IUGR	Repeat scan every 2 weeks if not delivered.
EFW	Below 10th birth weight percentile		Start antepartum surveillance and continue until delivery.
H/A ratio	In normal range		
Amniotic fluid volume	Low		Scan for anomalies, especially if IUGR present before 20 weeks. Amniocentesis indicated if IUGR is present before 20 weeks

*BPD = biparietal diameter; EFW = estimated fetal weight; H/A = head to abdominal ratio.

gain. Early dating should be performed in patients at increased risk for a fetus with IUGR. If IUGR has been diagnosed, fetal growth should be followed every 2 weeks until delivery using BPD, abdominal circumference, and estimated fetal weight, combined with assessment of the intrauterine environment. Timing of delivery will depend on fetal growth and antepartum surveillance. If there is no growth over a 2-week period, delivery is strongly recommended.

APPENDIX 10–1.

Crown-Rump Length*

Menstrual Maturity (weeks + days)	Crown-Rump Length (mm)		Menstrual Maturity (weeks + days)	Crown-Rump Length (mm)	
	Mean	2 SD		Mean	2 SD
6 + 2	7.0	3.3	10 + 0	33.0	7.2
6 + 3	6.5	1.4	10 + 1	33.8	7.6
6 + 4	7.0	4.6	10 + 2	35.2	7.3
6 + 5	6.5	4.2	10 + 3	36.0	7.9
6 + 6	10.0	2.6	10 + 4	37.3	9.7
			10 + 5	43.4	7.7
7 + 0	9.3	2.3	10 + 6	40.1	7.1
7 + 1	10.3	8.0			
7 + 2	11.8	5.7	11 + 0	46.7	6.1
7 + 3	12.8	4.8	11 + 1	43.6	7.2
7 + 4	13.4	6.7	11 + 2	47.5	6.2
7 + 5	15.4	3.6	11 + 3	48.8	5.9
7 + 6	15.4	4.4	11 + 4	49.0	9.5
			11 + 5	54.0	9.8
8 + 0	17.0	4.9	11 + 6	56.2	9.5
8 + 1	19.5	5.7			
8 + 2	19.4	6.2	12 + 0	58.3	9.4
8 + 3	20.4	5.0	12 + 1	56.8	7.2
8 + 4	21.3	3.8	12 + 2	59.4	6.6
8 + 5	20.9	2.4	12 + 3	62.6	8.6
8 + 6	23.2	3.6	12 + 4	63.5	9.5
			12 + 5	67.7	6.4
9 + 0	25.8	6.0	12 + 6	66.5	8.2
9 + 1	25.4	4.6			
9 + 2	26.7	4.4	13 + 0	72.5	4.2
9 + 3	27.0	2.8	13 + 1	69.7	8.5
9 + 4	32.5	4.2	13 + 2	73.0	15.1
9 + 5	30.0	10.0	13 + 3	77.0	8.5
9 + 6	31.3	5.5	13 + 4	—	—
			13 + 5	—	—
			13 + 6	76.0	5.7
			14 + 0	79.6	7.8

*Adapted from Robinson HP, Fleming JEE: A critical evaluation of sonar "crown-rump length" measurements. *Br J Obstet Gynaecol* 1975; 82:702.

APPENDIX 10–2.
Biparietal Diameter*

BPD (cm)	Menstrual Age (wk)	BPD (cm)	Menstrual Age (wk)	BPD (cm)	Menstrual Age (wk)	BPD (cm)	Menstrual Age (wk)
2.0	12.2	4.0	18.0	6.0	24.6	8.0	32.5
2.1	12.5	4.1	18.3	6.1	25.0	8.1	32.9
2.2	12.8	4.2	18.6	6.2	25.3	8.2	33.3
2.3	13.1	4.3	18.9	6.3	25.7	8.3	33.8
2.4	13.3	4.4	19.2	6.4	26.1	8.4	34.2
2.5	13.6	4.5	19.5	6.5	26.4	8.5	34.7
2.6	13.9	4.6	19.9	6.6	26.8	8.6	35.1
2.7	14.2	4.7	20.2	6.7	27.2	8.7	35.6
2.8	14.5	4.8	20.5	6.8	27.6	8.8	36.1
2.9	14.7	4.9	20.8	6.9	28.0	8.9	36.5
3.0	15.0	5.0	21.2	7.0	28.3	9.0	37.0
3.1	15.3	5.1	21.5	7.1	28.7	9.1	37.5
3.2	15.6	5.2	21.8	7.2	29.1	9.2	38.0
3.3	15.9	5.3	22.2	7.3	29.5	9.3	38.5
3.4	16.2	5.4	22.5	7.4	29.9	9.4	38.9
3.5	16.5	5.5	22.8	7.5	30.4	9.5	39.4
3.6	16.8	5.6	23.2	7.6	30.8	9.6	39.9
3.7	17.1	5.7	23.5	7.7	31.2	9.7	40.5
3.8	17.4	5.8	23.9	7.8	31.6	9.8	41.0
3.9	17.7	5.9	24.2	7.9	32.0	9.9	41.5
						10.0	42.0

*Adapted from Hadlock FP, Deter RL, Harrist RB: Fetal biparietal diameter. *J Ultrasound Med* 1982; 1:97–104.

APPENDIX 10–3.
Gestational Age Estimated From Femur Length (14 to 80 mm)*

Femur length (mm)	Jeanty			Hohler	Hadlock
	5th %ile†	50th %ile	95th %ile	50th %ile	50th %ile
14	11 + 5	13 + 6	16 + 1	13 + 1	13 + 6
15	12	14 + 1	16 + 3	13 + 4	14 + 1
16	12 + 3	14 + 4	16 + 6	13 + 6	14 + 4
17	12 + 5	14 + 6	17 + 1	14 + 1	14 + 6
18	13	15 + 1	17 + 3	14 + 4	15 + 1
19	13 + 3	15 + 4	17 + 6	14 + 6	15 + 3
20	13 + 5	15 + 6	18 + 1	15 + 1	15 + 5
21	14 + 1	16 + 2	18 + 4	15 + 4	16
22	14 + 3	16 + 4	18 + 6	15 + 6	16 + 2
23	14 + 5	16 + 6	19 + 1	16 + 1	16 + 4
24	15 + 1	17 + 2	19 + 4	16 + 4	16 + 6
25	15 + 3	17 + 4	19 + 6	16 + 6	17 + 1
26	15 + 6	18	20 + 1	17 + 1	17 + 4
27	16 + 1	18 + 2	20 + 4	17 + 4	17 + 6
28	16 + 4	18 + 5	20 + 6	17 + 6	18 + 1
29	16 + 6	19	21 + 1	18 + 2	18 + 4
30	17 + 1	19 + 3	21 + 4	18 + 4	18 + 6
31	17 + 4	19 + 6	22	19	19 + 1
32	17 + 6	20 + 1	22 + 2	19 + 3	19 + 4
33	18 + 2	20 + 4	22 + 5	19 + 5	19 + 6
34	18 + 5	20 + 6	23 + 1	20 + 1	20 + 2
35	19	21 + 1	23 + 3	20 + 4	20 + 5
36	19 + 3	21 + 4	23 + 6	20 + 6	21
37	19 + 6	22	24 + 1	21 + 2	21 + 3
38	20 + 1	22 + 3	24 + 4	21 + 5	21 + 6
39	20 + 4	22 + 5	24 + 6	22	22 + 1
40	20 + 6	23 + 1	25 + 2	22 + 3	22 + 4
41	21 + 2	23 + 4	25 + 5	22 + 6	22 + 6
42	21 + 5	23 + 6	26 + 1	23 + 1	23 + 2
43	22 + 1	24 + 2	26 + 4	23 + 4	23 + 5
44	22 + 4	24 + 5	26 + 6	24	24 + 1
45	22 + 6	25	27 + 1	24 + 4	24 + 4
46	23 + 1	25 + 3	27 + 4	24 + 6	24 + 6
47	23 + 4	25 + 6	28	25 + 2	25 + 2
48	24	26 + 1	28 + 3	25 + 5	25 + 5
49	24 + 3	26 + 4	28 + 6	26 + 1	26 + 1
50	24 + 6	27	29 + 1	26 + 4	26 + 4
51	25 + 1	27 + 3	29 + 4	27	27
52	25 + 4	27 + 6	30	27 + 3	27 + 3
53	26	28 + 1	30 + 3	27 + 6	27 + 6
54	26 + 3	28 + 4	30 + 6	28 + 2	28 + 1
55	26 + 6	29 + 1	31 + 2	28 + 5	28 + 5
56	27 + 2	29 + 4	31 + 5	29 + 1	29 + 1
57	27 + 5	29 + 6	32 + 1	29 + 4	29 + 4

Continued.

APPENDIX 10–3 (cont.).
Gestational Age Estimated From Femur Length (14 to 80 mm)*

Femur length (mm)	Jeanty 5th %ile†	Jeanty 50th %ile	Jeanty 95th %ile	Hohler 50th %ile	Hadlock 50th %ile
58	28 + 1	30 + 2	32 + 4	30 + 1	30
59	28 + 4	30 + 5	32 + 6	30 + 4	30 + 4
60	28 + 6	31 + 1	33 + 2	31	30 + 6
61	29 + 3	31 + 4	33 + 6	31 + 4	31 + 3
62	29 + 6	32	34 + 1	31 + 6	31 + 6
63	30 + 1	32 + 3	34 + 4	32 + 3	32 + 2
64	30 + 5	32 + 6	35 + 1	32 + 6	32 + 6
65	31 + 1	33 + 2	35 + 4	33 + 2	33 + 2
66	31 + 4	33 + 5	35 + 6	33 + 6	33 + 6
67	32	34 + 1	36 + 3	34 + 2	34 + 1
68	32 + 3	34 + 4	36 + 6	34 + 6	34 + 5
69	32 + 6	35	37 + 1	35 + 2	35 + 1
70	33 + 2	35 + 4	37 + 5	35 + 6	35 + 5
71	33 + 5	35 + 6	38 + 1	36 + 2	36 + 1
72	34 + 1	36 + 3	38 + 4	36 + 6	36 + 5
73	34 + 4	36 + 6	39	37 + 2	37 + 1
74	35 + 1	37 + 2	39 + 4	37 + 6	37 + 5
75	35 + 4	37 + 5	39 + 6	38 + 2	38 + 2
76	36	38 + 1	40 + 3	38 + 6	38 + 6
77	36 + 3	38 + 4	40 + 6	39 + 2	39 + 2
78	36 + 6	39 + 1	41 + 2	39 + 6	39 + 6
79	37 + 2	39 + 4	41 + 5	40 + 2	40 + 3
80	37 + 6	40	42 + 1	40 + 6	40 + 6

*Adapted from Jeanty P, Romero R: *Obstetrical Ultrasound.* New York, McGraw-Hill Book Co, 1984.
†Values expressed as whole plus fraction of weeks.

APPENDIX 10–4.
Gestational Age Estimated From Length of Humerus, Ulna, and Tibia*

Bone length (mm)	Humerus			Ulna			Tibia		
	5th %ile†	50th %ile	95th %ile	5th %ile	50th %ile	95th %ile	5th %ile	50th %ile	95th %ile
10	9 + 6	12 + 4	15 + 2	10 + 1	13 + 1	16 + 1	10 + 4	13 + 3	16 + 2
11	10 + 1	12 + 6	15 + 4	10 + 4	13 + 4	16 + 4	10 + 6	13 + 5	16 + 4
12	10 + 3	13 + 1	15 + 6	10 + 6	13 + 6	16 + 6	11 + 1	14 + 1	17
13	10 + 6	13 + 4	16 + 1	11 + 1	14 + 1	17 + 2	11 + 4	14 + 3	17 + 2
14	11 + 1	13 + 6	16 + 4	11 + 4	14 + 4	17 + 5	11 + 6	14 + 6	17 + 5
15	11 + 3	14 + 1	16 + 6	11 + 6	15	18	12 + 1	15 + 1	18
16	11 + 6	14 + 4	17 + 2	12 + 2	15 + 3	18 + 3	12 + 4	15 + 4	18 + 3
17	12 + 1	14 + 6	17 + 4	12 + 5	15 + 5	18 + 6	13	15 + 6	18 + 6
18	12 + 4	15 + 1	18	13 + 1	16 + 1	19 + 1	13 + 2	16 + 1	19 + 1
19	12 + 6	15 + 4	18 + 2	13 + 4	16 + 4	19 + 4	13 + 5	16 + 4	19 + 4
20	13 + 1	15 + 6	18 + 5	13 + 6	16 + 6	20	14 + 1	17	19 + 6
21	13 + 4	16 + 2	19 + 1	14 + 2	17 + 2	20 + 3	14 + 4	17 + 3	20 + 2
22	13 + 6	16 + 5	19 + 3	14 + 5	17 + 5	20 + 6	14 + 6	17 + 6	20 + 5
23	14 + 2	17 + 1	19 + 6	15 + 1	18 + 1	21 + 1	15 + 1	18 + 1	21 + 1
24	14 + 5	17 + 3	20 + 1	15 + 4	18 + 4	21 + 4	15 + 4	18 + 4	21 + 3
25	15 + 1	17 + 6	20 + 4	16	19	22 + 1	16	18 + 6	21 + 6
26	15 + 4	18 + 1	21	16 + 3	19 + 3	22 + 4	16 + 3	19 + 2	22 + 1
27	15 + 6	18 + 4	21 + 3	16 + 6	19 + 6	22 + 6	16 + 6	19 + 5	22 + 4
28	16 + 2	19	21 + 6	17 + 2	20 + 2	23 + 3	17 + 1	20 + 1	23
29	16 + 5	19 + 3	22 + 1	17 + 5	20 + 6	23 + 6	17 + 4	20 + 4	23 + 4
30	17 + 1	19 + 6	22 + 4	18 + 1	21 + 1	24 + 2	18 + 1	21	23 + 6
31	17 + 4	20 + 2	23	18 + 4	21 + 5	24 + 6	18 + 4	21 + 3	24 + 2
32	18	20 + 5	23 + 4	19 + 1	22 + 1	25 + 1	18 + 6	21 + 6	24 + 5
33	18 + 3	21 + 1	23 + 6	19 + 4	22 + 5	25 + 5	19 + 2	22 + 1	25 + 1
34	18 + 6	21 + 4	24 + 2	20 + 1	23 + 1	26 + 1	19 + 5	22 + 4	25 + 4
35	19 + 2	22	24 + 6	20 + 4	23 + 4	26 + 5	20 + 1	23 + 1	26

Continued.

APPENDIX 10–4 (cont.).
Gestational Age Estimated From Length of Humerus, Ulna, and Tibia*

Bone length (mm)	Humerus			Ulna			Tibia		
	5th %ile†	50th %ile	95th %ile	5th %ile	50th %ile	95th %ile	5th %ile	50th %ile	95th %ile
36	19 + 5	22 + 4	25 + 1	21 + 1	24 + 1	27 + 1	20 + 4	23 + 4	26 + 3
37	20 + 1	22 + 6	25 + 5	21 + 4	24 + 4	27 + 5	21	23 + 6	26 + 6
38	20 + 4	23 + 3	26 + 1	22 + 1	25 + 1	28 + 1	21 + 4	24 + 3	27 + 2
39	21 + 1	23 + 6	26 + 4	22 + 4	25 + 4	28 + 5	21 + 6	24 + 6	27 + 5
40	21 + 4	24 + 2	27 + 1	23 + 1	26 + 1	29 + 1	22 + 3	25 + 2	28 + 1
41	22	24 + 6	27 + 4	23 + 4	26 + 5	29 + 5	22 + 6	25 + 5	28 + 4
42	22 + 4	25 + 2	28	24 + 1	27 + 1	30 + 2	23 + 2	26 + 1	29 + 1
43	23	25 + 5	28 + 4	24 + 5	27 + 5	30 + 6	23 + 5	26 + 4	29 + 4
44	23 + 4	26 + 1	29	25 + 1	28 + 2	31 + 2	24 + 1	27 + 1	30
45	24	26 + 5	29 + 4	25 + 6	28 + 6	31 + 6	24 + 4	27 + 4	30 + 4
46	24 + 4	27 + 1	30	26 + 2	29 + 3	32 + 3	25 + 1	28	30 + 6
47	25	27 + 5	30 + 4	26 + 6	29 + 6	33	25 + 4	28 + 4	31 + 3
48	25 + 4	28 + 1	31	27 + 3	30 + 4	33 + 4	26 + 1	29	31 + 6
49	26	28 + 6	31 + 4	28	31 + 1	34 + 1	26 + 4	29 + 3	32 + 2
50	26 + 4	29 + 2	32	28 + 4	31 + 4	34 + 5	27	29 + 6	32 + 6
51	27 + 1	29 + 6	32 + 4	29 + 1	32 + 1	35 + 2	27 + 4	30 + 3	33 + 2
52	27 + 4	30 + 2	33 + 1	29 + 5	32 + 6	35 + 6	28	30 + 6	33 + 6
53	28 + 1	30 + 6	33 + 4	30 + 2	33 + 3	36 + 3	28 + 4	31 + 3	34 + 2
54	28 + 5	31 + 3	34 + 1	30 + 6	34	37	29	31 + 6	34 + 6
55	29 + 1	32	34 + 5	31 + 4	34 + 4	37 + 5	29 + 4	32 + 3	35 + 2
56	29 + 6	32 + 4	35 + 2	32 + 1	35 + 1	38 + 2	30	32 + 6	35 + 6
57	30 + 2	33 + 1	35 + 6	32 + 6	35 + 6	38 + 6	30 + 4	33 + 3	36 + 2
58	30 + 6	33 + 4	36 + 3	33 + 3	36 + 3	39 + 4	31	33 + 6	36 + 6
59	31 + 3	34 + 1	36 + 6	34	37 + 1	40 + 1	31 + 4	34 + 3	37 + 2

60	32	34 + 6	37 + 4	34 + 4	37 + 5	40 + 6	32	34 + 6	37 + 6
61	32 + 4	35 + 2	38 + 1	35 + 2	38 + 2	41 + 3	32 + 4	35 + 3	38 + 2
62	33 + 1	35 + 6	38 + 5	35 + 6	39	42	33	35 + 6	38 + 6
63	33 + 6	36 + 4	39 + 2	36 + 4	39 + 4	42 + 5	33 + 4	36 + 4	39 + 3
64	34 + 3	37 + 1	39 + 6	37 + 1	40 + 2	43 + 2	34 + 1	37	39 + 6
65	35	37 + 5	40 + 4				34 + 4	37 + 4	40 + 3
66	35 + 4	38 + 2	41 + 1				35 + 1	38	41
67	36 + 1	38 + 6	41 + 5				35 + 5	38 + 4	41 + 4
68	36 + 6	39 + 4	42 + 2				36 + 1	39 + 1	42
69	37 + 3	40 + 1	42 + 6				36 + 6	39 + 5	42 + 4

*Adapted from Jeanty P, Romero R: *Obstetrical Ultrasound.* New York, McGraw-Hill Book Co, 1984.
†Values expressed as whole plus fraction of weeks.

APPENDIX 10–5.

Biparietal Diameter and Weeks Gestation Predicted From Inner and Outer Orbital Diameters*†

BPD (cm)	Gestation (wk)	IOD (cm)	OOD (cm)	BPD (cm)	Gestation (wk)	IOD (cm)	OOD (cm)
1.9	11.6	0.5	1.3	5.8	24.3	1.6	4.1
2.0	11.6	0.5	1.4	5.9	24.3	1.6	4.2
2.1	12.1	0.6	1.5	6.0	24.7	1.6	4.3
2.2	12.6	0.6	1.6	6.1	25.2	1.6	4.3
2.3	12.6	0.6	1.7	6.2	25.2	1.6	4.4
2.4	13.1	0.7	1.7	6.3	25.7	1.7	4.4
2.5	13.6	0.7	1.8	6.4	26.2	1.7	4.5
2.6	13.6	0.7	1.9	6.5	26.2	1.7	4.5
2.7	14.1	0.8	2.0	6.6	26.7	1.7	4.6
2.8	14.6	0.8	2.1	6.7	27.2	1.7	4.6
2.9	14.6	0.8	2.1	6.8	27.6	1.7	4.7
3.0	15.0	0.9	2.2	6.9	28.1	1.7	4.7
3.1	15.5	0.9	2.3	7.0	28.6	1.8	4.8
3.2	15.5	0.9	2.4	7.1	29.1	1.8	4.8
3.3	16.0	1.0	2.5	7.3	29.6	1.8	4.9
3.4	16.5	1.0	2.5	7.4	30.0	1.8	5.0
3.5	16.5	1.0	2.6	7.5	30.6	1.8	5.0
3.6	17.0	1.0	2.7	7.6	31.0	1.8	5.1
3.7	17.5	1.1	2.7	7.7	31.5	1.8	5.1
3.8	17.9	1.1	2.8	7.8	32.0	1.8	5.2
4.0	18.4	1.2	3.0	7.9	32.5	1.9	5.2
4.2	18.9	1.2	3.1	8.0	33.0	1.9	5.3
4.3	19.4	1.2	3.2	8.2	33.5	1.9	5.4
4.4	19.4	1.3	3.2	8.3	34.0	1.9	5.4
4.5	19.9	1.3	3.3	8.4	34.4	1.9	5.4
4.6	20.4	1.3	3.4	8.5	35.0	1.9	5.5
4.7	20.4	1.3	3.4	8.6	35.4	1.9	5.5
4.8	20.9	1.4	3.5	8.8	35.9	1.9	5.6
4.9	21.3	1.4	3.6	8.9	36.4	1.9	5.6
5.0	21.3	1.4	3.6	9.0	36.9	1.9	5.7
5.1	21.8	1.4	3.7	9.1	37.3	1.9	5.7
5.2	22.3	1.4	3.8	9.2	37.8	1.9	5.8
5.3	22.3	1.5	3.8	9.3	38.3	1.9	5.8
5.4	22.8	1.5	3.9	9.4	38.8	1.9	5.8
5.5	23.3	1.5	4.0	9.6	39.3	1.9	5.9
5.6	23.3	1.5	4.0	9.7	39.8	1.9	5.9
5.7	23.8	1.5	4.1				

*Adapted from Mayden KL, Tortora M, Berkowitz RL, et al: *Am J Obstet Gynecol* 1982; 144:289.
†IOD = inner orbital diameter; OOD = outer orbital diameter.

APPENDIX 10–6.

Head-to-Abdominal Circumference Ratio*†

Menstrual Age (wk)	No. of Measurements	H/A Circumference Ratio		
		5th %ile	Mean	95th %ile
13–14	18	1.14	1.23	1.31
15–16	39	1.05	1.22	1.39
17–18	77	1.07	1.18	1.29
19–20	54	1.09	1.18	1.26
21–22	41	1.06	1.15	1.25
23–24	22	1.05	1.13	1.21
25–26	18	1.04	1.13	1.22
27–28	36	1.05	1.13	1.22
29–30	23	0.99	1.10	1.21
31–32	31	0.96	1.07	1.17
33–34	42	0.96	1.04	1.11
35–36	49	0.93	1.02	1.11
37–38	67	0.92	0.98	1.05
39–40	47	0.87	0.97	1.06
41–42	4	0.93	0.96	1.00

*Adapted from Campbell S, Thoms A: *Br J Obstet Gynecol* 1977; 84:165.
†Mean fetal H/A circumference ratios with 5th and 95th percentile limits related to menstrual age from 13 to 42 weeks; values have been combined into 2-week groups to smooth out fluctuations due to small numbers (568 individual measurements).

APPENDIX 10–7.

Fetal Weight Estimated From Biparietal Diameter and Abdominal Circumference*†

BPD (cm)	Abdominal Circumference (cm)											
	15.5	16.0	16.5	17.0	17.5	18.0	18.5	19.0	19.5	20.0	20.5	21.0
3.1	224	234	244	255	267	279	291	304	318	332	346	362
3.2	231	241	251	263	274	286	299	312	326	340	355	371
3.3	237	248	259	270	282	294	307	321	335	349	365	381
3.4	244	255	266	278	290	302	316	329	344	359	374	391
3.5	251	262	274	285	298	311	324	338	353	368	384	401
3.6	259	270	281	294	306	319	333	347	362	378	394	411
3.7	266	278	290	302	315	328	342	357	372	388	404	422
3.8	274	286	298	310	324	337	352	366	382	398	415	432
3.9	282	294	306	319	333	347	361	376	392	409	426	444
4.0	290	303	315	328	342	356	371	386	403	419	437	455
4.1	299	311	324	338	352	366	381	397	413	430	448	467
4.2	308	320	333	347	361	376	392	408	424	442	460	479
4.3	317	330	343	357	371	387	402	419	436	453	472	491
4.4	326	339	353	367	382	397	413	430	447	465	484	504
4.5	335	349	363	377	393	408	425	442	459	478	497	517
4.6	345	359	373	388	404	420	436	454	472	490	510	530
4.7	355	369	384	399	415	431	448	466	484	503	523	544
4.8	366	380	395	410	426	443	460	478	497	517	537	558
4.9	376	391	406	422	438	455	473	491	510	530	551	572
5.0	387	402	418	434	451	468	486	505	524	544	565	587

Continued.

APPENDIX 10–7 (cont.).

Fetal Weight Estimated From Biparietal Diameter and Abdominal Circumference*†

BPD	Abdominal Circumference (cm)											
(cm)	15.5	16.0	16.5	17.0	17.5	18.0	18.5	19.0	19.5	20.0	20.5	21.0
5.1	399	414	430	446	463	481	499	518	538	559	580	602
5.2	410	426	442	459	476	494	513	532	552	573	595	618
5.3	422	438	455	472	489	508	527	547	567	589	611	634
5.4	435	451	468	485	503	522	541	561	582	604	627	650
5.5	447	464	481	499	517	536	556	577	598	620	643	667
5.6	461	477	495	513	532	551	571	592	614	636	660	684
5.7	474	491	509	527	547	566	587	608	630	653	677	701
5.8	488	505	524	542	562	582	603	625	647	670	695	719
5.9	502	520	539	558	578	598	619	642	664	688	713	738
6.0	517	535	554	573	594	615	636	659	682	706	731	757
6.1	532	550	570	590	610	632	654	677	700	725	750	777
6.2	547	566	586	606	627	649	672	695	719	744	770	797
6.3	563	583	603	624	645	667	690	714	738	764	790	817
6.4	580	600	620	641	663	686	709	733	758	784	811	838
6.5	597	617	638	659	682	705	728	753	778	805	832	860
6.6	614	635	656	678	701	724	748	773	799	826	853	882
6.7	632	653	675	697	720	744	769	794	820	848	876	905
6.8	651	672	694	717	740	765	790	816	842	870	898	928
6.9	670	691	714	737	761	786	811	838	865	893	922	952
7.0	689	711	734	758	782	807	833	860	888	916	946	976
7.1	709	732	755	779	804	830	856	883	912	941	971	1,002
7.2	730	763	777	801	827	853	880	907	936	965	996	1,027
7.3	751	775	799	824	850	876	904	932	961	991	1,022	1,054
7.4	773	797	822	847	874	901	928	957	987	1,017	1,049	1,081
7.5	796	820	845	871	898	925	954	983	1,013	1,044	1,076	1,109
7.6	819	844	870	896	923	951	980	1,009	1,040	1,072	1,104	1,137
7.7	843	868	894	921	949	977	1,007	1,037	1,068	1,100	1,133	1,167
7.8	868	894	920	947	975	1,004	1,034	1,065	1,096	1,129	1,162	1,197
7.9	893	919	946	974	1,003	1,032	1,062	1,094	1,126	1,159	1,193	1,228
8.0	919	946	973	1,002	1,031	1,061	1,091	1,123	1,156	1,189	1,224	1,259
8.1	946	973	1,001	1,030	1,060	1,090	1,121	1,153	1,187	1,221	1,256	1,292
8.2	974	1,001	1,030	1,059	1,089	1,120	1,152	1,185	1,218	1,253	1,288	1,325
8.3	1,002	1,030	1,059	1,089	1,120	1,151	1,183	1,217	1,251	1,286	1,322	1,359
8.4	1,032	1,060	1,090	1,120	1,151	1,183	1,216	1,249	1,284	1,320	1,356	1,394
8.5	1,062	1,091	1,121	1,151	1,183	1,216	1,249	1,283	1,318	1,355	1,392	1,430
8.6	1,093	1,122	1,153	1,184	1,216	1,249	1,283	1,318	1,354	1,390	1,428	1,467
8.7	1,125	1,155	1,186	1,218	1,250	1,284	1,318	1,353	1,390	1,427	1,465	1,505
8.8	1,157	1,188	1,220	1,252	1,285	1,319	1,354	1,390	1,427	1,465	1,504	1,543
8.9	1,191	1,222	1,254	1,287	1,321	1,356	1,391	1,428	1,465	1,503	1,543	1,583
9.0	1,226	1,258	1,290	1,324	1,358	1,393	1,429	1,456	1,504	1,543	1,583	1,624
9.1	1,262	1,294	1,327	1,361	1,396	1,432	1,468	1,506	1,544	1,584	1,624	1,666
9.2	1,299	1,332	1,365	1,400	1,435	1,471	1,508	1,546	1,586	1,626	1,667	1,709
9.3	1,337	1,370	1,404	1,439	1,475	1,512	1,550	1,588	1,628	1,668	1,710	1,753
9.4	1,376	1,410	1,444	1,480	1,516	1,554	1,592	1,631	1,671	1,712	1,755	1,798
9.5	1,416	1,450	1,486	1,522	1,559	1,597	1,635	1,675	1,716	1,758	1,800	1,844
9.6	1,457	1,492	1,528	1,565	1,602	1,641	1,680	1,720	1,762	1,804	1,847	1,892

9.7	1,500	1,535	1,572	1,609	1,647	1,686	1,726	1,767	1,809	1,852	1,895	1,940
9.8	1,544	1,580	1,617	1,654	1,693	1,733	1,773	1,815	1,857	1,900	1,945	1,990
9.9	1,589	1,625	1,663	1,701	1,740	1,781	1,822	1,864	1,907	1,951	1,996	2,042
10.0	1,635	1,672	1,710	1,749	1,789	1,830	1,871	1,914	1,958	2,002	2,048	2,094

BPD	Abdominal Circumference (cm)												
(cm)	21.5	22.0	22.5	23.0	23.5	24.0	24.5	25.0	25.5	26.0	26.5	27.0	27.5
3.1	378	395	412	431	450	470	491	513	536	559	584	610	638
3.2	388	405	423	441	461	481	502	525	548	572	597	624	651
3.3	397	415	433	452	472	493	514	537	560	585	611	638	666
3.4	408	425	444	463	483	504	526	549	573	598	624	652	680
3.5	418	436	455	475	495	517	539	562	587	612	638	666	695
3.6	429	447	466	486	507	529	552	575	600	626	653	681	710
3.7	440	458	478	498	519	542	565	589	614	640	667	696	725
3.8	451	470	490	510	532	554	578	602	628	654	682	711	741
3.9	462	482	502	523	545	568	592	616	642	669	697	727	757
4.0	474	494	514	536	558	581	606	631	657	684	713	743	773
4.1	486	506	527	549	572	595	620	645	672	700	729	759	790
4.2	498	519	540	562	585	609	634	660	688	716	745	776	807
4.3	511	532	554	576	600	624	649	676	703	732	762	793	825
4.4	524	545	567	590	614	639	665	692	719	749	779	810	843
4.5	538	559	581	605	629	654	680	708	736	765	796	828	861
4.6	551	573	596	620	644	670	696	724	753	783	814	846	880
4.7	565	588	611	635	660	686	713	741	770	801	832	865	899
4.8	580	602	626	650	676	702	730	758	788	819	851	884	919
4.9	594	617	641	666	692	719	747	776	806	837	870	903	938
5.0	610	633	657	683	709	736	765	794	824	856	889	923	959
5.1	625	649	674	699	726	754	783	812	843	876	909	944	980
5.2	641	665	690	717	744	772	801	831	863	895	929	964	1,001
5.3	657	682	708	734	762	790	820	851	883	916	950	986	1,023
5.4	674	699	725	752	780	809	839	870	903	936	971	1,007	1,045
5.5	691	717	743	771	799	828	859	891	924	958	993	1,030	1,068
5.6	709	735	762	789	818	848	879	911	945	979	1,015	1,052	1,091
5.7	727	753	780	809	838	869	900	933	966	1,001	1,038	1,075	1,114
5.8	745	772	800	829	858	889	921	954	989	1,024	1,061	1,099	1,139
5.9	764	792	820	849	879	911	943	977	1,011	1,047	1,085	1,123	1,163
6.0	784	811	840	870	900	932	965	999	1,035	1,071	1,109	1,148	1,189
6.1	804	832	861	891	922	955	988	1,023	1,058	1,095	1,134	1,173	1,214
6.2	824	853	882	913	945	977	1,011	1,046	1,083	1,120	1,159	1,199	1,241
6.3	845	874	904	935	967	1,001	1,035	1,071	1,107	1,145	1,185	1,226	1,268
6.4	867	896	927	958	991	1,025	1,059	1,096	1,133	1,171	1,211	1,253	1,295
6.5	889	919	950	982	1,015	1,049	1,084	1,121	1,159	1,198	1,238	1,280	1,323
6.6	911	942	973	1,006	1,039	1,074	1,110	1,147	1,185	1,225	1,266	1,308	1,352
6.7	935	965	997	1,030	1,065	1,100	1,136	1,174	1,213	1,253	1,294	1,337	1,381
6.8	958	990	1,022	1,056	1,090	1,126	1,163	1,201	1,241	1,281	1,323	1,367	1,411
6.9	983	1,015	1,048	1,082	1,117	1,153	1,190	1,229	1,269	1,310	1,353	1,397	1,442
7.0	1,008	1,040	1,074	1,108	1,144	1,181	1,219	1,258	1,298	1,340	1,383	1,427	1,473

Continued.

APPENDIX 10–7 (cont.).
Fetal Weight Estimated From Biparietal Diameter and Abdominal Circumference*†

BPD (cm)	Abdominal Circumference (cm)												
	21.5	22.0	22.5	23.0	23.5	24.0	24.5	25.0	25.5	26.0	26.5	27.0	27.5
7.1	1,033	1,066	1,100	1,135	1,171	1,209	1,247	1,287	1,328	1,370	1,414	1,459	1,505
7.2	1,060	1,093	1,128	1,163	1,200	1,238	1,277	1,317	1,358	1,401	1,445	1,491	1,538
7.3	1,087	1,121	1,156	1,192	1,229	1,267	1,307	1,348	1,390	1,433	1,478	1,524	1,571
7.4	1,114	1,149	1,184	1,221	1,259	1,297	1,338	1,379	1,421	1,465	1,511	1,557	1,605
7.5	1,143	1,178	1,214	1,251	1,289	1,328	1,369	1,411	1,454	1,499	1,544	1,592	1,640
7.6	1,172	1,207	1,244	1,281	1,320	1,360	1,401	1,444	1,487	1,533	1,579	1,627	1,676
7.7	1,202	1,238	1,275	1,313	1,352	1,393	1,434	1,477	1,522	1,567	1,614	1,663	1,712
7.8	1,232	1,269	1,306	1,345	1,385	1,426	1,468	1,512	1,557	1,603	1,650	1,699	1,749
7.9	1,264	1,301	1,339	1,378	1,418	1,460	1,503	1,547	1,592	1,639	1,687	1,737	1,787
8.0	1,296	1,333	1,372	1,412	1,453	1,495	1,538	1,583	1,629	1,676	1,725	1,775	1,826
8.1	1,329	1,367	1,406	1,446	1,488	1,531	1,575	1,620	1,666	1,714	1,763	1,814	1,866
8.2	1,363	1,401	1,441	1,482	1,524	1,567	1,612	1,657	1,704	1,753	1,803	1,854	1,906
8.3	1,397	1,436	1,477	1,518	1,561	1,605	1,650	1,696	1,744	1,793	1,843	1,895	1,948
8.4	1,433	1,473	1,513	1,555	1,599	1,643	1,689	1,735	1,784	1,833	1,884	1,936	1,990
8.5	1,469	1,510	1,551	1,594	1,637	1,682	1,728	1,776	1,825	1,875	1,926	1,979	2,033
8.6	1,507	1,548	1,589	1,633	1,677	1,722	1,769	1,817	1,866	1,917	1,969	2,022	2,077
8.7	1,545	1,586	1,629	1,673	1,717	1,764	1,811	1,859	1,909	1,960	2,013	2,067	2,122
8.8	1,584	1,626	1,669	1,714	1,759	1,806	1,854	1,903	1,953	2,005	2,058	2,113	2,169
8.9	1,625	1,667	1,711	1,756	1,802	1,849	1,897	1,947	1,998	2,050	2,104	2,159	2,216
9.0	1,666	1,709	1,753	1,799	1,845	1,893	1,942	1,992	2,044	2,097	2,151	2,207	2,264
9.1	1,708	1,752	1,797	1,843	1,890	1,938	1,988	2,039	2,091	2,144	2,199	2,255	2,313
9.2	1,752	1,796	1,841	1,888	1,936	1,984	2,035	2,086	2,139	2,193	2,248	2,305	2,363
9.3	1,796	1,841	1,887	1,934	1,982	2,032	2,083	2,135	2,188	2,242	2,298	2,356	2,414
9.4	1,842	1,887	1,934	1,982	2,030	2,080	2,132	2,184	2,238	2,293	2,350	2,407	2,467
9.5	1,889	1,935	1,982	2,030	2,080	2,130	2,182	2,235	2,289	2,345	2,402	2,460	2,520
9.6	1,937	1,984	2,031	2,080	2,130	2,181	2,233	2,287	2,342	2,398	2,456	2,515	2,575
9.7	1,986	2,033	2,082	2,131	2,181	2,233	2,286	2,340	2,396	2,452	2,510	2,570	2,631
9.8	2,037	2,085	2,133	2,183	2,234	2,286	2,340	2,395	2,451	2,508	2,567	2,627	2,688
9.9	2,089	2,137	2,186	2,237	2,288	2,341	2,395	2,450	2,507	2,565	2,624	2,684	2,746
10.0	2,142	2,191	2,241	2,292	2,344	2,397	2,452	2,507	2,564	2,623	2,682	2,743	2,806

BPD (cm)	Abdominal Circumference (cm)											
	28.0	28.5	29.0	29.5	30.0	30.5	31.0	31.5	32.0	32.5	33.0	33.5
3.1	666	696	726	759	793	828	865	903	943	985	1,029	1,075
3.2	680	710	742	774	809	844	882	921	961	1,004	1,048	1,094
3.3	695	725	757	790	825	861	899	938	979	1,022	1,067	1,114
3.4	710	740	773	806	841	878	916	956	998	1,041	1,087	1,134
3.5	725	756	789	823	858	896	934	975	1,017	1,061	1,107	1,154
3.6	740	772	805	840	876	913	953	993	1,036	1,080	1,127	1,175
3.7	756	788	822	857	893	931	971	1,012	1,056	1,101	1,147	1,196
3.8	772	805	839	874	911	950	990	1,032	1,076	1,121	1,168	1,218
3.9	789	822	856	892	930	969	1,009	1,052	1,096	1,142	1,190	1,240

4.0	806	839	874	911	949	988	1,029	1,072	1,117	1,163	1,212	1,262
4.1	828	857	892	929	968	1,008	1,049	1,093	1,138	1,185	1,234	1,285
4.2	841	875	911	948	987	1,028	1,070	1,114	1,159	1,207	1,256	1,308
4.3	859	893	930	968	1,007	1,048	1,091	1,135	1,181	1,229	1,279	1,331
4.4	877	912	949	987	1,027	1,069	1,112	1,157	1,204	1,252	1,303	1,355
4.5	896	932	969	1,008	1,048	1,090	1,134	1,179	1,226	1,275	1,326	1,380
4.6	915	951	989	1,028	1,069	1,112	1,156	1,202	1,249	1,299	1,351	1,404
4.7	934	971	1,010	1,049	1,091	1,134	1,178	1,225	1,273	1,323	1,375	1,430
4.8	954	992	1,031	1,071	1,113	1,156	1,201	1,248	1,297	1,348	1,401	1,455
4.9	975	1,013	1,052	1,093	1,135	1,179	1,225	1,272	1,322	1,373	1,426	1,482
5.0	996	1,034	1,074	1,115	1,158	1,203	1,249	1,297	1,347	1,399	1,452	1,508
5.1	1,017	1,056	1,096	1,138	1,181	1,226	1,273	1,322	1,372	1,425	1,479	1,535
5.2	1,039	1,078	1,119	1,161	1,205	1,251	1,298	1,347	1,398	1,451	1,506	1,563
5.3	1,061	1,101	1,142	1,185	1,229	1,276	1,323	1,373	1,425	1,478	1,533	1,591
5.4	1,084	1,124	1,166	1,209	1,254	1,301	1,349	1,399	1,452	1,506	1,562	1,620
5.5	1,107	1,148	1,190	1,234	1,279	1,327	1,376	1,426	1,479	1,534	1,590	1,649
5.6	1,131	1,172	1,215	1,259	1,305	1,353	1,402	1,454	1,507	1,562	1,619	1,678
5.7	1,155	1,197	1,240	1,285	1,332	1,380	1,430	1,482	1,535	1,591	1,649	1,709
5.8	1,180	1,222	1,266	1,311	1,358	1,407	1,458	1,510	1,564	1,621	1,679	1,739
5.9	1,205	1,248	1,292	1,338	1,386	1,435	1,486	1,539	1,594	1,651	1,710	1,770
6.0	1,231	1,274	1,319	1,366	1,414	1,464	1,515	1,569	1,624	1,682	1,741	1,802
6.1	1,257	1,301	1,346	1,393	1,442	1,493	1,545	1,599	1,655	1,713	1,773	1,835
6.2	1,284	1,328	1,374	1,422	1,471	1,522	1,575	1,630	1,686	1,745	1,805	1,868
6.3	1,311	1,356	1,403	1,451	1,501	1,552	1,606	1,661	1,718	1,777	1,838	1,901
6.4	1,339	1,385	1,432	1,481	1,531	1,583	1,637	1,693	1,751	1,810	1,872	1,935
6.5	1,368	1,414	1,462	1,511	1,562	1,615	1,669	1,725	1,784	1,844	1,906	1,970
6.6	1,397	1,444	1,492	1,542	1,594	1,647	1,702	1,759	1,817	1,878	1,941	2,006
6.7	1,427	1,474	1,523	1,574	1,626	1,679	1,735	1,792	1,852	1,913	1,976	2,042
6.8	1,458	1,505	1,555	1,606	1,658	1,713	1,769	1,827	1,887	1,949	2,012	2,078
6.9	1,489	1,537	1,587	1,639	1,692	1,747	1,803	1,862	1,922	1,985	2,049	2,116
7.0	1,521	1,570	1,620	1,672	1,726	1,781	1,839	1,898	1,959	2,022	2,087	2,154
7.1	1,553	1,603	1,654	1,706	1,761	1,817	1,875	1,934	1,996	2,059	2,125	2,193
7.2	1,586	1,636	1,688	1,741	1,796	1,853	1,911	1,971	2,044	2,098	2,164	2,232
7.3	1,620	1,671	1,723	1,777	1,832	1,890	1,948	2,009	2,072	2,137	2,203	2,272
7.4	1,655	1,706	1,759	1,813	1,869	1,927	1,987	2,048	2,111	2,176	2,244	2,313
7.5	1,690	1,742	1,795	1,850	1,907	1,965	2,025	2,087	2,151	2,217	2,265	2,354
7.6	1,727	1,779	1,833	1,888	1,945	2,004	2,065	2,127	2,192	2,258	2,326	2,397
7.7	1,764	1,816	1,871	1,927	1,985	2,044	2,105	2,168	2,233	2,300	2,369	2,440
7.8	1,801	1,855	1,910	1,966	2,025	2,085	2,146	2,210	2,275	2,343	2,412	2,484
7.9	1,840	1,894	1,949	2,006	2,065	2,126	2,188	2,252	2,318	2,386	2,456	2,528
8.0	1,879	1,934	1,990	2,048	2,107	2,168	2,231	2,296	2,362	2,431	2,501	2,574
8.1	1,919	1,975	2,031	2,089	2,149	2,211	2,275	2,340	2,407	2,476	2,547	2,620
8.2	1,960	2,016	2,073	2,132	2,193	2,255	2,319	2,385	2,462	2,522	2,594	2,667
8.3	2,002	2,059	2,116	2,176	2,237	2,300	2,364	2,431	2,499	2,569	2,641	2,715
8.4	2,045	2,102	2,160	2,220	2,282	2,345	2,410	2,477	2,546	2,617	2,689	2,764
8.5	2,089	2,146	2,205	2,266	2,328	2,392	2,457	2,525	2,594	2,665	2,739	2,814
8.6	2,134	2,192	2,251	2,312	2,375	2,439	2,505	2,573	2,643	2,715	2,789	2,864
8.7	2,179	2,238	2,298	2,359	2,423	2,488	2,554	2,623	2,693	2,765	2,840	2,916
8.8	2,226	2,285	2,346	2,408	2,472	2,537	2,604	2,673	2,744	2,817	2,892	2,968
8.9	2,274	2,333	2,394	2,457	2,521	2,587	2,655	2,725	2,796	2,869	2,944	3,021
9.0	2,322	2,382	2,444	2,507	2,572	2,639	2,707	2,777	2,849	2,923	2,998	3,076

Continued.

APPENDIX 10–7 (cont.).
Fetal Weight Estimated From Biparietal Diameter and Abdominal Circumference*†

BPD (cm)	Abdominal Circumference (cm)											
	28.0	28.5	29.0	29.5	30.0	30.5	31.0	31.5	32.0	32.5	33.0	33.5
9.1	2,372	2,433	2,495	2,559	2,624	2,691	2,760	2,830	2,903	2,977	3,053	3,131
9.2	2,423	2,484	2,547	2,611	2,677	2,744	2,814	2,885	2,958	3,032	3,109	3,187
9.3	2,475	2,536	2,599	2,664	2,731	2,799	2,869	2,940	3,014	3,089	3,166	3,245
9.4	2,527	2,590	2,653	2,719	2,786	2,854	2,925	2,997	3,070	3,146	3,224	3,303
9.5	2,582	2,644	2,709	2,774	2,842	2,911	2,982	3,054	3,129	3,205	3,283	3,362
9.6	2,637	2,700	2,765	2,831	2,899	2,969	3,040	3,113	3,188	3,264	3,343	3,423
9.7	2,693	2,757	2,822	2,889	2,958	3,028	3,099	3,173	3,248	3,325	3,404	3,484
9.8	2,751	2,815	2,881	2,948	3,017	3,088	3,160	3,234	3,309	3,387	3,466	3,547
9.9	2,810	2,874	2,941	3,009	3,078	3,149	3,222	3,296	3,372	3,450	3,529	3,611
10.0	2,870	2,935	3,002	3,070	3,140	3,211	3,285	3,359	3,436	3,514	3,594	3,676

BPD (cm)	Abdominal Circumference (cm)												
	34.0	34.5	35.0	35.5	36.0	36.5	37.0	37.5	38.0	38.5	39.0	39.5	40.0
3.1	1,123	1,173	1,225	1,279	1,336	1,396	1,458	1,523	1,591	1,661	1,735	1,812	1,893
3.2	1,143	1,193	1,246	1,301	1,358	1,418	1,481	1,546	1,615	1,686	1,761	1,838	1,920
3.3	1,163	1,214	1,267	1,323	1,381	1,441	1,504	1,570	1,639	1,711	1,786	1,865	1,946
3.4	1,183	1,235	1,289	1,345	1,403	1,464	1,528	1,595	1,664	1,737	1,812	1,891	1,973
3.5	1,204	1,256	1,311	1,367	1,426	1,488	1,552	1,619	1,689	1,762	1,839	1,918	2,001
3.6	1,226	1,278	1,333	1,390	1,450	1,512	1,577	1,645	1,715	1,789	1,865	1,945	2,029
3.7	1,247	1,300	1,356	1,413	1,474	1,536	1,602	1,670	1,741	1,815	1,893	1,973	2,057
3.8	1,269	1,323	1,379	1,437	1,498	1,561	1,627	1,696	1,768	1,842	1,920	2,001	2,086
3.9	1,292	1,346	1,402	1,461	1,523	1,586	1,653	1,722	1,794	1,870	1,948	2,030	2,115
4.0	1,315	1,369	1,426	1,486	1,548	1,612	1,679	1,749	1,822	1,898	1,977	2,059	2,145
4.1	1,338	1,393	1,451	1,511	1,573	1,638	1,706	1,776	1,849	1,926	2,005	2,088	2,174
4.2	1,361	1,417	1,475	1,536	1,599	1,664	1,733	1,804	1,878	1,954	2,035	2,118	2,205
4.3	1,385	1,442	1,500	1,562	1,625	1,691	1,760	1,832	1,906	1,984	2,064	2,148	2,236
4.4	1,410	1,467	1,526	1,588	1,652	1,718	1,788	1,860	1,935	2,013	2,094	2,179	2,267
4.5	1,435	1,492	1,552	1,614	1,679	1,746	1,816	1,889	1,964	2,043	2,125	2,210	2,298
4.6	1,460	1,518	1,579	1,641	1,706	1,774	1,845	1,918	1,994	2,073	2,156	2,241	2,330
4.7	1,486	1,545	1,605	1,669	1,734	1,803	1,874	1,948	2,024	2,104	2,187	2,273	2,363
4.8	1,512	1,571	1,633	1,697	1,763	1,832	1,904	1,978	2,055	2,136	2,219	2,306	2,396
4.9	1,539	1,599	1,661	1,725	1,792	1,861	1,934	2,009	2,086	2,167	2,251	2,339	2,429
5.0	1,566	1,626	1,689	1,754	1,821	1,891	1,964	2,040	2,118	2,200	2,284	2,372	2,463
5.1	1,594	1,655	1,718	1,783	1,851	1,922	1,995	2,071	2,150	2,232	2,317	2,406	2,498
5.2	1,622	1,683	1,747	1,813	1,882	1,953	2,027	2,103	2,183	2,266	2,351	2,440	2,532
5.3	1,651	1,713	1,777	1,843	1,913	1,984	2,059	2,136	2,216	2,299	2,386	2,475	2,568
5.4	1,680	1,742	1,807	1,874	1,944	2,016	2,091	2,169	2,250	2,333	2,420	2,510	2,604
5.5	1,710	1,773	1,838	1,906	1,976	2,049	2,124	2,203	2,284	2,368	2,456	2,546	2,640
5.6	1,740	1,803	1,869	1,938	2,008	2,082	2,158	2,237	2,319	2,403	2,491	2,582	2,677
5.7	1,770	1,835	1,901	1,970	2,041	2,115	2,192	2,272	2,354	2,439	2,528	2,619	2,714
5.8	1,802	1,866	1,934	2,003	2,075	2,150	2,227	2,307	2,390	2,475	2,564	2,657	2,752
5.9	1,834	1,899	1,966	2,037	2,109	2,184	2,262	2,342	2,426	2,512	2,602	2,694	2,790
6.0	1,866	1,932	2,000	2,071	2,144	2,219	2,298	2,379	2,463	2,550	2,640	2,733	2,829
6.1	1,899	1,965	2,034	2,105	2,179	2,255	2,334	2,416	2,500	2,588	2,678	2,772	2,869
6.2	1,932	1,999	2,069	2,140	2,215	2,291	2,371	2,453	2,538	2,626	2,717	2,811	2,909

6.3	1,967	2,034	2,104	2,176	2,251	2,328	2,408	2,491	2,577	2,665	2,757	2,851	2,949
6.4	2,001	2,069	2,140	2,213	2,288	2,366	2,446	2,530	2,616	2,705	2,797	2,892	2,991
6.5	2,037	2,105	2,176	2,250	2,326	2,404	2,485	2,569	2,656	2,745	2,838	2,933	3,032
6.6	2,073	2,142	2,213	2,287	2,364	2,443	2,524	2,609	2,696	2,786	2,879	2,975	3,075
6.7	2,109	2,179	2,251	2,326	2,403	2,482	2,564	2,649	2,737	2,827	2,921	3,018	3,117
6.8	2,147	2,217	2,290	2,365	2,442	2,522	2,605	2,690	2,778	2,869	2,964	3,061	3,161
6.9	2,184	2,255	2,329	2,404	2,482	2,563	2,646	2,732	2,821	2,912	3,007	3,104	3,205
7.0	2,223	2,295	2,368	2,444	2,523	2,604	2,688	2,774	2,863	2,955	3,050	3,149	3,250
7.1	2,262	2,334	2,409	2,485	2,564	2,646	2,730	2,817	2,907	2,999	3,095	3,193	3,295
7.2	2,302	2,375	2,450	2,527	2,607	2,689	2,773	2,861	2,951	3,044	3,140	3,239	3,341
7.3	2,343	2,416	2,491	2,569	2,649	2,732	2,817	2,905	2,996	3,089	3,186	3,285	3,388
7.4	2,384	2,458	2,534	2,612	2,693	2,776	2,862	2,950	3,041	3,135	3,232	3,332	3,435
7.5	2,426	2,501	2,577	2,656	2,737	2,821	2,907	2,996	3,088	3,182	3,279	3,380	3,483
7.6	2,469	2,544	2,621	2,700	2,782	2,866	2,953	3,042	3,134	3,229	3,327	3,428	3,531
7.7	2,513	2,588	2,666	2,746	2,828	2,912	3,000	3,090	3,182	3,277	3,376	3,477	3,581
7.8	2,557	2,633	2,711	2,792	2,874	2,959	3,047	3,137	3,230	3,326	3,425	3,526	3,631
7.9	2,603	2,679	2,757	2,838	2,921	3,007	3,095	3,186	3,279	3,376	3,475	3,576	3,681
8.0	2,649	2,725	2,804	2,886	2,969	3,056	3,144	3,235	3,329	3,426	3,525	3,627	3,733
8.1	2,695	2,773	2,852	2,934	3,018	3,105	3,194	3,286	3,380	3,477	3,577	3,679	3,785
8.2	2,743	2,821	2,901	2,983	3,068	3,155	3,244	3,336	3,431	3,529	3,629	3,732	3,838
8.3	2,791	2,870	2,950	3,033	3,118	3,206	3,296	3,388	3,483	3,581	3,682	3,785	3,891
8.4	2,841	2,920	3,001	3,084	3,169	3,257	3,348	3,441	3,536	3,634	3,735	3,839	3,945
8.5	2,891	2,970	3,052	3,135	3,221	3,310	3,401	3,494	3,590	3,688	3,790	3,894	4,000
8.6	2,942	3,022	3,104	3,188	3,274	3,363	3,454	3,548	3,644	3,743	3,845	3,949	4,056
8.7	2,994	3,074	3,157	3,241	3,328	3,417	3,509	3,603	3,700	3,799	3,901	4,005	4,113
8.8	3,047	3,128	3,210	3,295	3,383	3,472	3,565	3,659	3,756	3,855	3,958	4,063	4,170
8.9	3,101	3,182	3,265	3,351	3,438	3,528	3,621	3,716	3,813	3,913	4,015	4,120	4,228
9.0	3,155	3,237	3,321	3,407	3,495	3,585	3,678	3,773	3,871	3,971	4,074	4,179	4,287
9.1	3,211	3,293	3,377	3,464	3,552	3,643	3,736	3,832	3,930	4,030	4,133	4,239	4,347
9.2	3,268	3,350	3,435	3,522	3,611	3,702	3,795	3,891	3,989	4,090	4,193	4,299	4,408
9.3	3,326	3,409	3,494	3,581	3,670	3,761	3,855	3,951	4,050	4,151	4,254	4,361	4,469
9.4	3,384	3,468	3,553	3,641	3,738	3,822	3,916	4,013	4,111	4,213	4,316	4,423	4,532
9.5	3,444	3,528	3,614	3,701	3,791	3,884	3,978	4,075	4,174	4,275	4,379	4,486	4,595
9.6	3,505	3,589	3,675	3,763	3,854	3,946	4,041	4,138	4,237	4,339	4,443	4,550	4,659
9.7	3,567	3,651	3,738	3,826	3,917	4,010	4,105	4,202	4,302	4,404	4,508	4,615	4,724
9.8	3,630	3,715	3,802	3,890	3,981	4,074	4,170	4,267	4,367	4,469	4,573	4,680	4,790
9.9	3,694	3,779	3,866	3,956	4,047	4,140	4,236	4,333	4,433	4,536	4,640	4,747	4,857
10.0	3,759	3,845	3,932	4,022	4,113	4,207	4,303	4,400	4,501	4,603	4,708	4,815	4,924

Adapted from Shepard MJ, Richards VA, Berkowitz RL, et al: An evaluation of two equations for predicting fetal weight by ultrasound. *Am J Obstet Gynecol* 1982; 142:47.
SD = ±106.0 gm/kg birth weight.

APPENDIX 10–8.
Fetal Weight Estimated from Abdominal Circumference and Femur Length*

Femur Length (cm)	Abdominal Circumference (cm)																				
	20.0	20.5	21.0	21.5	22.0	22.5	23.0	23.5	24.0	24.5	25.0	25.5	26.0	26.5	27.0	27.5	28.0	28.5	29.0	29.5	30.0
4.0	663	691	720	751	783	816	851	887	925	964	1,006	1,048	1,093	1,139	1,188	1,239	1,291	1,346	1,403	1,463	1,525
4.1	680	709	738	769	802	836	871	907	946	986	1,027	1,070	1,115	1,162	1,211	1,262	1,315	1,371	1,429	1,489	1,551
4.2	697	726	757	788	821	855	891	928	967	1,007	1,049	1,093	1,138	1,186	1,235	1,287	1,340	1,396	1,454	1,515	1,578
4.3	715	745	776	808	841	875	912	949	988	1,029	1,071	1,116	1,162	1,209	1,259	1,311	1,365	1,422	1,480	1,541	1,605
4.4	734	764	795	827	861	896	933	971	1,010	1,051	1,094	1,139	1,185	1,234	1,284	1,336	1,391	1,448	1,507	1,568	1,632
4.5	753	783	815	847	882	917	954	993	1,033	1,074	1,118	1,163	1,210	1,259	1,309	1,362	1,417	1,474	1,534	1,596	1,660
4.6	772	803	835	868	903	939	976	1,015	1,056	1,098	1,142	1,187	1,235	1,284	1,335	1,388	1,444	1,501	1,561	1,623	1,688
4.7	792	823	856	889	924	961	999	1,038	1,079	1,122	1,166	1,212	1,260	1,310	1,361	1,415	1,471	1,529	1,589	1,652	1,717
4.8	812	844	877	911	947	984	1,022	1,062	1,103	1,146	1,191	1,237	1,286	1,336	1,388	1,442	1,498	1,557	1,618	1,681	1,746
4.9	833	865	899	933	969	1,007	1,046	1,086	1,128	1,171	1,216	1,263	1,312	1,363	1,415	1,470	1,527	1,585	1,647	1,710	1,776
5.0	855	887	921	956	993	1,031	1,070	1,111	1,153	1,197	1,243	1,290	1,339	1,390	1,443	1,498	1,555	1,615	1,676	1,740	1,806
5.1	877	910	944	980	1,016	1,055	1,095	1,136	1,179	1,223	1,269	1,317	1,367	1,418	1,471	1,527	1,584	1,644	1,706	1,770	1,837
5.2	899	933	967	1,004	1,041	1,080	1,120	1,162	1,205	1,250	1,296	1,344	1,395	1,447	1,500	1,556	1,614	1,674	1,737	1,801	1,868
5.3	922	956	992	1,028	1,066	1,105	1,146	1,188	1,232	1,277	1,324	1,373	1,423	1,476	1,530	1,586	1,645	1,705	1,768	1,833	1,900
5.4	946	981	1,016	1,053	1,091	1,131	1,172	1,215	1,259	1,305	1,352	1,401	1,452	1,505	1,560	1,617	1,675	1,736	1,799	1,865	1,933
5.5	971	1,005	1,041	1,079	1,118	1,158	1,199	1,242	1,287	1,333	1,381	1,431	1,482	1,535	1,591	1,648	1,707	1,768	1,832	1,897	1,966
5.6	995	1,031	1,067	1,105	1,144	1,185	1,227	1,271	1,316	1,362	1,411	1,461	1,513	1,566	1,622	1,679	1,739	1,801	1,864	1,931	1,999
5.7	1,021	1,057	1,094	1,132	1,172	1,213	1,255	1,299	1,345	1,392	1,441	1,491	1,544	1,598	1,654	1,712	1,772	1,834	1,898	1,964	2,033
5.8	1,047	1,084	1,121	1,160	1,200	1,242	1,285	1,329	1,375	1,422	1,472	1,523	1,575	1,630	1,686	1,744	1,805	1,867	1,932	1,999	2,068
5.9	1,074	1,111	1,149	1,188	1,229	1,271	1,314	1,359	1,406	1,454	1,503	1,555	1,608	1,663	1,719	1,778	1,839	1,902	1,966	2,034	2,103
6.0	1,102	1,139	1,178	1,217	1,258	1,301	1,345	1,390	1,437	1,485	1,535	1,587	1,641	1,696	1,753	1,812	1,873	1,936	2,002	2,069	2,139
6.1	1,130	1,168	1,207	1,247	1,289	1,331	1,376	1,421	1,469	1,518	1,568	1,620	1,674	1,730	1,788	1,847	1,908	1,972	2,038	2,105	2,175
6.2	1,160	1,198	1,237	1,278	1,319	1,363	1,408	1,454	1,501	1,551	1,602	1,654	1,709	1,765	1,823	1,882	1,944	2,008	2,074	2,142	2,212
6.3	1,189	1,228	1,268	1,309	1,351	1,395	1,440	1,487	1,535	1,585	1,636	1,689	1,744	1,800	1,858	1,919	1,981	2,045	2,111	2,180	2,250
6.4	1,220	1,259	1,299	1,341	1,384	1,428	1,473	1,520	1,569	1,619	1,671	1,724	1,779	1,836	1,895	1,956	2,018	2,082	2,149	2,218	2,289

6.5	1,251	1,291	1,332	1,373	1,417	1,461	1,507	1,555	1,604	1,655	1,707	1,760	1,816	1,873	1,932	1,993	2,056	2,121	2,188	2,256	2,328
6.6	1,284	1,324	1,365	1,407	1,451	1,496	1,542	1,590	1,640	1,691	1,743	1,797	1,853	1,911	1,970	2,031	2,094	2,160	2,227	2,296	2,367
6.7	1,317	1,357	1,399	1,441	1,486	1,531	1,578	1,626	1,676	1,728	1,780	1,835	1,891	1,949	2,009	2,070	2,134	2,199	2,267	2,336	2,408
6.8	1,351	1,391	1,433	1,477	1,521	1,567	1,615	1,663	1,713	1,765	1,819	1,873	1,930	1,988	2,048	2,110	2,174	2,240	2,307	2,377	2,449
6.9	1,385	1,427	1,469	1,513	1,558	1,604	1,652	1,701	1,752	1,804	1,857	1,913	1,970	2,028	2,089	2,151	2,215	2,281	2,348	2,418	2,490
7.0	1,421	1,463	1,506	1,550	1,595	1,642	1,690	1,740	1,791	1,843	1,897	1,953	2,010	2,069	2,130	2,192	2,256	2,322	2,391	2,461	2,533
7.1	1,458	1,500	1,543	1,588	1,633	1,681	1,729	1,779	1,830	1,883	1,938	1,994	2,051	2,110	2,171	2,234	2,299	2,365	2,433	2,504	2,576
7.2	1,495	1,538	1,581	1,626	1,673	1,720	1,769	1,819	1,871	1,924	1,979	2,035	2,093	2,153	2,214	2,277	2,342	2,408	2,477	2,547	2,620
7.3	1,534	1,577	1,621	1,666	1,713	1,761	1,810	1,861	1,913	1,966	2,021	2,078	2,136	2,196	2,258	2,321	2,386	2,453	2,521	2,592	2,665
7.4	1,573	1,616	1,661	1,707	1,754	1,802	1,852	1,903	1,955	2,009	2,065	2,122	2,180	2,240	2,302	2,365	2,431	2,498	2,566	2,637	2,710
7.5	1,614	1,657	1,702	1,749	1,796	1,845	1,895	1,946	1,999	2,053	2,109	2,166	2,225	2,285	2,347	2,411	2,476	2,543	2,612	2,683	2,756
7.6	1,655	1,699	1,745	1,791	1,839	1,888	1,939	1,990	2,043	2,098	2,154	2,211	2,270	2,331	2,393	2,457	2,523	2,590	2,659	2,730	2,803
7.7	1,698	1,742	1,788	1,835	1,883	1,933	1,983	2,035	2,089	2,144	2,200	2,258	2,317	2,378	2,440	2,504	2,570	2,638	2,707	2,778	2,851
7.8	1,741	1,786	1,833	1,880	1,928	1,978	2,029	2,082	2,135	2,191	2,247	2,305	2,365	2,426	2,488	2,553	2,618	2,686	2,755	2,827	2,899
7.9	1,786	1,832	1,878	1,926	1,975	2,025	2,076	2,129	2,183	2,238	2,295	2,353	2,413	2,474	2,537	2,602	2,668	2,735	2,805	2,876	2,949
8.0	1,832	1,878	1,925	1,973	2,022	2,073	2,124	2,177	2,232	2,287	2,344	2,403	2,463	2,524	2,587	2,652	2,718	2,785	2,855	2,926	2,999
8.1	1,879	1,926	1,973	2,021	2,071	2,121	2,173	2,227	2,281	2,337	2,394	2,453	2,513	2,575	2,638	2,702	2,769	2,837	2,906	2,977	3,050
8.2	1,928	1,974	2,022	2,070	2,120	2,171	2,224	2,277	2,332	2,388	2,446	2,504	2,565	2,626	2,690	2,754	2,821	2,889	2,958	3,029	3,202
8.3	1,978	2,024	2,072	2,121	2,171	2,223	2,275	2,329	2,384	2,440	2,498	2,557	2,617	2,679	2,743	2,807	2,874	2,942	3,011	3,082	3,155

Continued.

APPENDIX 10–8 (cont.).
Fetal Weight Estimated from Abdominal Circumference and Femur Length*

Femur Length (cm)	Abdominal Circumference (cm)																			
	30.5	31.0	31.5	32.0	32.5	33.0	33.5	34.0	34.5	35.0	35.5	36.0	36.5	37.0	37.5	38.0	38.5	39.0	39.5	40.0
4.0	1,590	1,658	1,729	1,802	1,879	1,959	2,042	2,129	2,220	2,314	2,413	2,515	2,622	2,734	2,850	2,972	3,098	3,230	3,367	3,511
4.1	1,617	1,685	1,756	1,830	1,907	1,987	2,071	2,158	2,249	2,344	2,442	2,545	2,652	2,764	2,880	3,002	3,128	3,260	3,397	3,540
4.2	1,644	1,712	1,783	1,858	1,935	2,016	2,100	2,187	2,279	2,373	2,472	2,575	2,683	2,794	2,911	3,032	3,159	3,290	3,427	3,570
4.3	1,671	1,740	1,812	1,886	1,964	2,045	2,129	2,217	2,308	2,404	2,503	2,606	2,713	2,825	2,942	3,063	3,189	3,321	3,458	3,600
4.4	1,699	1,768	1,840	1,915	1,993	2,075	2,159	2,247	2,339	2,434	2,533	2,637	2,744	2,856	2,973	3,094	3,220	3,352	3,488	3,630
4.5	1,727	1,797	1,869	1,944	2,023	2,105	2,189	2,278	2,370	2,465	2,565	2,668	2,776	2,888	3,004	3,125	3,251	3,383	3,519	3,661
4.6	1,756	1,826	1,898	1,974	2,053	2,135	2,220	2,309	2,401	2,497	2,596	2,700	2,807	2,919	3,036	3,157	3,283	3,414	3,550	3,692
4.7	1,785	1,855	1,928	2,004	2,084	2,166	2,251	2,340	2,432	2,528	2,628	2,732	2,840	2,952	3,068	3,189	3,315	3,446	3,582	3,723
4.8	1,814	1,885	1,959	2,035	2,115	2,197	2,283	2,372	2,464	2,560	2,660	2,764	2,872	2,984	3,100	3,221	3,347	3,478	3,613	3,754
4.9	1,845	1,916	1,990	2,066	2,146	2,229	2,315	2,404	2,497	2,593	2,693	2,797	2,905	3,017	3,133	3,254	3,380	3,510	3,645	3,786
5.0	1,875	1,947	2,021	2,098	2,178	2,261	2,347	2,437	2,530	2,626	2,726	2,830	2,938	3,050	3,166	3,287	3,412	3,542	3,677	3,818
5.1	1,906	1,978	2,053	2,130	2,210	2,294	2,380	2,470	2,563	2,659	2,760	2,864	2,972	3,084	3,200	3,320	3,445	3,575	3,710	3,850
5.2	1,938	2,010	2,085	2,163	2,243	2,327	2,413	2,503	2,597	2,693	2,794	2,898	3,006	3,117	3,234	3,354	3,479	3,608	3,743	3,882
5.3	1,970	2,043	2,118	2,196	2,277	2,360	2,447	2,537	2,631	2,728	2,828	2,932	3,040	3,152	3,268	3,388	3,513	3,642	3,776	3,915
5.4	2,003	2,076	2,151	2,229	2,311	2,395	2,482	2,572	2,665	2,762	2,863	2,967	3,075	3,186	3,302	3,422	3,547	3,676	3,809	3,948
5.5	2,036	2,109	2,185	2,264	2,345	2,429	2,516	2,607	2,700	2,797	2,898	3,002	3,110	3,221	3,337	3,457	3,581	3,710	3,843	3,981
5.6	2,070	2,143	2,220	2,298	2,380	2,464	2,552	2,642	2,736	2,833	2,933	3,038	3,145	3,257	3,372	3,492	3,616	3,744	3,877	4,015
5.7	2,104	2,178	2,254	2,333	2,415	2,500	2,587	2,678	2,772	2,869	2,970	3,074	3,181	3,293	3,408	3,527	3,651	3,779	3,911	4,048
5.8	2,139	2,213	2,290	2,369	2,451	2,536	2,624	2,714	2,808	2,905	3,006	3,110	3,218	3,329	3,444	3,563	3,686	3,814	3,946	4,082
5.9	2,175	2,249	2,326	2,405	2,488	2,573	2,660	2,751	2,845	2,942	3,043	3,147	3,254	3,366	3,480	3,599	3,722	3,849	3,981	4,117
6.0	2,211	2,286	2,363	2,442	2,525	2,610	2,698	2,789	2,883	2,980	3,080	3,184	3,292	3,403	3,517	3,636	3,758	3,885	4,016	4,151
6.1	2,248	2,323	2,400	2,480	2,562	2,647	2,736	2,827	2,921	3,018	3,118	3,222	3,329	3,440	3,554	3,673	3,795	3,921	4,052	4,186
6.2	2,285	2,360	2,438	2,518	2,600	2,686	2,774	2,865	2,959	3,056	3,157	3,260	3,367	3,478	3,592	3,710	3,832	3,957	4,087	4,222
6.3	2,323	2,398	2,476	2,556	2,639	2,725	2,813	2,904	2,998	3,095	3,195	3,299	3,406	3,516	3,630	3,747	3,869	3,994	4,124	4,257
6.4	2,362	2,437	2,515	2,595	2,678	2,764	2,852	2,943	3,037	3,134	3,235	3,338	3,445	3,555	3,668	3,785	3,906	4,031	4,160	4,293

6.5	2,401	2,477	2,555	2,635	2,718	2,804	2,892	2,983	3,077	3,174	3,274	3,378	3,484	3,594	3,707	3,824	3,944	4,069	4,197	4,329
6.6	2,441	2,517	2,595	2,675	2,759	2,844	2,933	3,024	3,118	3,215	3,315	3,418	3,524	3,633	3,746	3,863	3,983	4,106	4,234	4,366
6.7	2,481	2,557	2,636	2,716	2,800	2,885	2,974	3,065	3,159	3,256	3,355	3,458	3,564	3,673	3,786	3,902	4,021	4,144	4,271	4,402
6.8	2,523	2,599	2,677	2,758	2,841	2,927	3,016	3,107	3,200	3,297	3,397	3,499	3,605	3,714	3,826	3,941	4,060	4,183	4,309	4,439
6.9	2,564	2,641	2,719	2,800	2,884	2,969	3,058	3,149	3,242	3,339	3,438	3,541	3,646	3,754	3,866	3,981	4,100	4,222	4,347	4,477
7.0	2,607	2,683	2,762	2,843	2,927	3,012	3,101	3,192	3,285	3,381	3,481	3,583	3,688	3,796	3,907	4,022	4,140	4,261	4,386	4,514
7.1	2,650	2,727	2,806	2,887	2,970	3,056	3,144	3,235	3,328	3,424	3,523	3,625	3,730	3,838	3,948	4,062	4,180	4,300	4,425	4,552
7.2	2,694	2,771	2,850	2,931	3,014	3,100	3,188	3,279	3,372	3,468	3,567	3,668	3,772	3,880	3,990	4,104	4,220	4,340	4,464	4,591
7.3	2,739	2,816	2,895	2,976	3,059	3,145	3,233	3,323	3,416	3,512	3,610	3,712	3,816	3,922	4,032	4,145	4,261	4,381	4,503	4,629
7.4	2,785	2,861	2,940	3,021	3,105	3,190	3,278	3,369	3,461	3,557	3,655	3,756	3,859	3,966	4,075	4,187	4,303	4,421	4,543	4,668
7.5	2,831	2,908	2,987	3,068	3,151	3,236	3,324	3,414	3,507	3,602	3,700	3,800	3,903	4,009	4,118	4,230	4,344	4,462	4,583	4,708
7.6	2,878	2,955	3,034	3,115	3,198	3,283	3,371	3,461	3,553	3,648	3,745	3,845	3,948	4,053	4,161	4,272	4,387	4,504	4,624	4,747
7.7	2,926	3,003	3,081	3,162	3,245	3,331	3,418	3,508	3,600	3,694	3,791	3,891	3,993	4,098	4,205	4,316	4,429	4,545	4,665	4,787
7.8	2,974	3,051	3,130	3,211	3,294	3,379	3,466	3,555	3,647	3,741	3,838	3,937	4,039	4,143	4,250	4,360	4,472	4,588	4,706	4,827
7.9	3,024	3,100	3,179	3,260	3,343	3,427	3,514	3,604	3,695	3,789	3,885	3,984	4,085	4,188	4,295	4,404	4,515	4,630	4,748	4,868
8.0	3,074	3,151	3,229	3,310	3,392	3,477	3,564	3,653	3,744	3,837	3,933	4,031	4,131	4,234	4,340	4,448	4,559	4,673	4,790	4,909
8.1	3,125	3,202	3,280	3,360	3,443	3,527	3,614	3,702	3,793	3,886	3,981	4,079	4,179	4,281	4,386	4,493	4,604	4,716	4,832	4,950
8.2	3,177	3,253	3,332	3,412	3,494	3,578	3,664	3,752	3,843	3,935	4,030	4,127	4,226	4,328	4,432	4,539	4,648	4,760	4,875	4,992
8.3	3,230	3,306	3,384	3,464	3,546	3,630	3,716	3,803	3,893	3,985	4,080	4,176	4,275	4,376	4,479	4,585	4,693	4,804	4,918	5,034

*Adapted from Hadlock FP, Harrist RB, Carpenter RJ, et al: *Radiology* 1984; 150:535.

REFERENCES

1. Calvert JP, Crean EE, Newcombe RG, et al: Antenatal screening by measurement of symphysis-fundus height. *Br Med J* 1982; 205:846.
2. Villar J, Belizán JM: The timing factor in the pathophysiology of the intrauterine growth retardation syndrome. *Obstet Gynecol Surv* 1982; 37:499.
3. Robinson HP: Sonar measurement of fetal crown-rump length as a means of assessing maturity in first trimester of pregnancy. *Br Med J* 1973; 4:28.
4. Robinson HP, Flemming JEE: A critical evaluation of sonar "crown-rump length" measurements. *Br J Obstet Gynaecol* 1975; 82:702.
5. Campbell S, Dewhurst CJ: Diagnosis of the small for dates fetus by serial ultrasound cephalometry. *Lancet* 1971; 2:1001.
6. Campbell S, Thoms A: Ultrasound measurement of the fetal head to abdomen circumference ratio in the assessment of growth retardation. *Br J Obstet Gynaecol* 1977; 84:165.
7. Hadlock FP, Deter RL, Carpenter RJ, et al: Estimating fetal age: Effect of head shape on BPD. *Am. J Roentgenol* 1981; 137:83.
8. Deter RL, Harrist RB, Hadlock FP, et al: Fetal head and abdominal circumference. II: A critical re-evaluation of the relationship to menstrual age. *JCU* 1982; 10:365.
9. Mayden KL, Tortora M, Berkowitz RL, et al: Orbital diameters: A new parameter for prenatal diagnosis and dating. *Am J Obstet Gynecol* 1982; 144:289.
10. O'Brien GD, Queenan JT: Growth of the ultrasound fetal femur length during normal pregnancy. *Am J Obstet Gynecol* 1981; 141:833.
11. O'Brien GD, Queenan JT, Campbell S: Assessment of gestational age in the second trimester by real-time ultrasound measurement of the femur length. *Am J Obstet Gynecol* 1981; 139:540.
12. Jeanty P, Romero R: *Obstetrical Ultrasound*. New York, McGraw-Hill Book Co, 1984.
13. Campbell S, Wilkin D: Ultrasonic measurement of fetal abdomen circumference in the estimation of fetal weight. *Br J Obstet Gynaecol* 1975; 82:689.
14. Evans MI, Mukherjee AB, Shulman JD: Animal models of intrauterine growth retardation. *Obstet Gynecol Surv* 1983; 38:183.
15. Shepard MJ, Richards VA, Berkowitz RL, et al: An evaluation of two equations for predicting fetal weight by ultrasound. *Am J Obstet Gynecol* 1982; 142:47.
16. Hadlock FP, Harrist RB, Carpenter RJ, et al: Sonographic estimation of fetal weight. *Radiology* 1984; 150:535.
17. Ott WJ, Doyle S: Ultrasonic diagnosis of altered fetal growth by use of a normal ultrasonic fetal weight curve. *Obstet Gynecol* 1984; 63:201.
18. Lubchenco LC, Hansman C, Dressler M, et al: Intrauterine growth as estimated from liveborn birth weight data at 24 to 42 weeks of gestation. *J Pediatr* 1963; 32:793.
19. Campbell S, Thoms A: ULtrasound measurement of the fetal head-to-abdomen circumference ratio in the assessment of growth retardation. *Br J Obstet Gynaecol* 1977; 84:165.
20. Crane JP, Kopta M: Prediction of intrauterine growth retardation via ultrasonographically measured head to abdomen circumference ratios. *Obstet Gynecol* 1979; 54:597.

21. Chinn DH, Bolding DB, Callen PW, et al: Ultrasonographic identification of fetal lower extremity epiphyseal ossification centers. *Radiology* 1983; 147:815.
22. Gentili P, Trasimeni A, Giorlandino C: Fetal ossification centers as predictors of gestational age in normal and abnormal pregnancies. *J Ultrasound Med* 1984; 3:193.
23. Manning FA, Hill LM, Platt LD: Qualitative amniotic fluid volume determination by ultrasound: Antepartum detection of intrauterine growth retardation. *Am J Obstet Gynecol* 1981; 139:254.
24. Mercer LJ, Brown LG, Petres RE, et al: A survey of pregnancies complicated by decreased amniotic fluid. *Am J Obstet Gynecol* 1984; 149:355.
25. Grannum PAT, Berkowitz RL, Hobbins JC: The ultrasonic changes in the maturing placenta and their relation to fetal pulmonic maturity. *Am J Obstet Gynecol* 1979; 133:915.
26. Levine LR: *Placental grades and gestational age* (thesis). Yale University School of Medicine, New Haven, Conn, March 1981.
27. Kazzi GM, Gross TL, Sokol RJ, et al: Detection of intrauterine growth retardation: A new use of sonographic placental grading. *Am J Obstet Gynecol* 1983; 145:733.
28. Griffin D, Cohen-Overbeck T, Campbell S: Fetal and uteroplacental blood flow. *Clin Obstet Gynecol* 1983; 10(3):565.
29. Brosen I, Dixon HG, Robertson WB: Fetal growth retardation and the arteries of the placental bed. *Br J Obstet Gynaecol* 1977; 84:656.
30. Shepard BL, Bonnar J: An ultrastructural study of uteroplacental spiral arteries in hypertensive and normotensive pregnancies and fetal growth retardation. *Br J Obstet Gynaecol* 1981; 88:695.
31. Fleischer A, Schulman H, Farmakides G, et al: Umbilical artery velocity waveforms and intrauterine growth retardation. *Am J Obstet Gynecol* 1985; 151:502.
32. McCowan LM, Erskine LA, Ritchie K: Umbilical artery doppler blood flow studies in the preterm small for gestational age fetus. *Am J Obstet Gynecol* 1987; 156:655.
33. Fleischer A, Anyaegbunam AA, Schulman H, et al: Uterine and umbilical artery velocimetry during normal labor. *Am J Obstet Gynecol* 1987; 157:40.

11

Doppler Blood Flow and Fetal Growth Retardation

Steven L. Warsof, M.D.
Donald L. Levy, M.D.

To most physicians ultrasonic imaging connotes a real-time, two-dimensional picture enabling the scanner to visualize the fetus in utero. This use of real-time ultrasound to monitor fetal growth is discussed in detail in Chapter 10. Ultrasound, however, can also be used with Doppler principles of motion detection to quantitate blood flow. These techniques are widely used in vascular laboratories to study blood flow in peripheral arteries and veins and have replaced more invasive studies such as angiography.

As fetal growth is dependent on maternal blood flow to the uterus to provide nutrients and fetal blood flow to the placenta to obtain these nutrients and clear its metabolic wastes, it seems logical that abnormalities in these flows could be the physiologic basis of fetal abnormalities. Prior to Doppler techniques, flow studies in human fetuses were limited because of their invasive nature. Because ultrasound uses nonionizing energy, which has no known biologic hazards to the fetus, many investigators are now applying Doppler methods to study fetal blood flow, growth, and well-being.

It is the purpose of this chapter to review the principles, techniques, and limitations of Doppler flow studies and how they have been used to detect fetal abnormalities.

DOPPLER PRINCIPLES

The first reports of the use of Doppler ultrasound for measurement of fetal blood velocity wave forms and flow were described in the late 1970s.[1,2] The Doppler principle involves a change in the ultrasound frequency when it interfaces with a moving object. In this case there is an increase in ultrasonic frequency when blood is flowing toward the ultrasonic beam. With the development of directional Doppler systems, flow toward the ultrasound beam giving a positive Doppler shift can be differentiated from flow away from the beam, which gives a negative Doppler shift.

Continuous-Wave Doppler Systems

Initially, studies involved low-intensity, continuous-wave Doppler systems similar to those used to detect fetal heart rates. The continuous-wave system involved two piezoelectric crystals, one continuously transmitting, the other receiving ultrasound signals. This system had two major deficiencies. First, the technique was blind in that fetal vessels were not visualized and vessels were identified only by a characteristic audio signal. Second, the ultrasound beam frequency crossed several vessels, and an entire spectrum of signals was created from these different vessels (Fig 11–1).

Pulsed-Wave Doppler Systems

Pulsed gated ultrasound overcame some of the deficiencies of the continuous-wave system. In the pulsed-wave units a single piezoelectric crystal was used to both transmit and receive. Short bursts of ultrasound were emitted and electronically timed so that only returning signals from a specified depth of penetration, or gate, would be received. This gate could be adjusted by the operator.

MEASUREMENT OF FETAL BLOOD FLOW

Blood velocity can be measured by the Doppler shift as noted in equation 1.

$$V = 1/2\frac{c\Delta f}{f_o\cos\theta} \qquad (1)$$

where V = velocity, f_o = transmitting frequency (2,000 to 4,000 kHz), c = velocity of sound in soft tissue (1,540 m/sec), θ = angle of insonation, and Δf = Doppler shift (kHz). Blood flow is related to this velocity as shown in equation 2.

$$Q = V \cdot A = \frac{V\pi d^2}{4} \qquad (2)$$

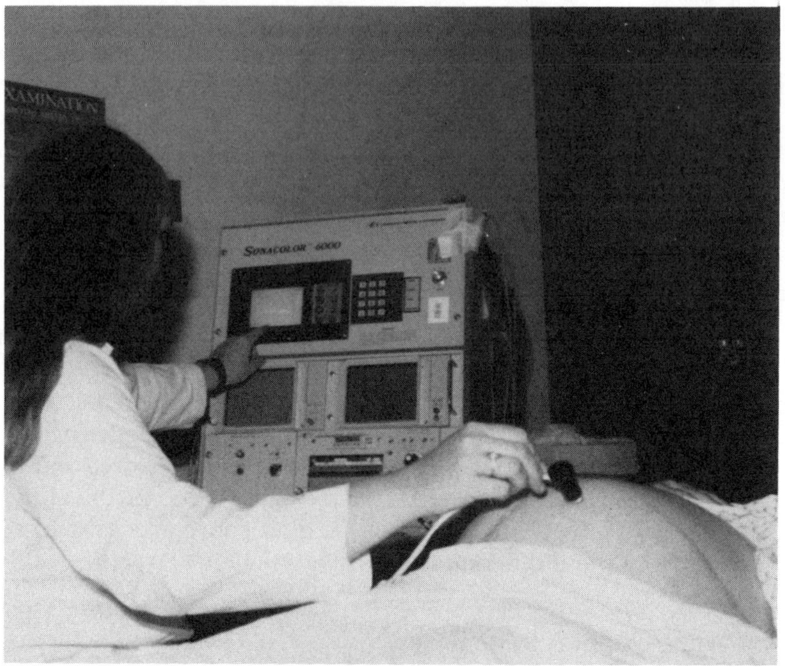

FIG 11–1.
Continuous-wave Doppler system (Sonacolor 6000, Carolina Medical Electronics, Inc., King, N.C.).

where Q = blood flow, V = blood velocity, A = cross-sectional area, and d = vessel diameter.

Measurement of blood flow therefore became dependent on the measurement of three variables: the Doppler shift frequency, the angle of insonation, and the diameter of the vessel to be measured. Inasmuch as blood flow is frequently expressed per kilogram body weight, a fourth variable, fetal weight, needs to be determined.

The Doppler shift frequencies can be measured with respect to time by computerized fast Fourier transformations. With this technique the data can be expressed and stored audibly on magnetic tape or visually on a cathode ray tube or strip chart as the flow velocity wave form (FVWF).

The angle of insonation, vessel diameter, and fetal weight cannot be determined by Doppler scans alone. The development of duplex ultrasound systems, which combine real-time ultrasound with a pulsed Doppler system, allows all of these measurements and blood flow to be measured by one ultrasound machine.[3,4]

Using this combined system a real-time scan can be performed in which the vessel whose flow is to be measured can be visualized. The Doppler beam can be aimed at the vessel and the pulsed Doppler gate placed precisely in the center or across the diameter of the vessel. The angle can be determined with precision and the vessel diameter likewise measured. This technology was quickly applied to determine blood velocity and flow in the umbilical artery, vein, fetal thoracic and abdominal aortas, and maternal uterine vessels.[5–7]

Errors in Fetal Blood Flow Measurements

Major discrepancies in these studies were quickly realized.[8] The reader is referred to Griffin et al.[5] for detailed analysis of these discrepancies. Aside from the Doppler shift frequencies, each of the measured parameters introduced a major error in the calculation. Perhaps the largest error was introduced in measuring the vessel diameter. Because vessel diameters vary from 4 to 8 mm, an error of even 1 mm could represent as much as 25% variation. This error was compounded because flow was proportional to the diameter of the vessel squared. The angle of insonation was also at best crudely measured. Because flow is inversely proportional to $\cos\theta$, a few degrees of error, especially when the angle of insonation became increasingly acute, could make a major difference in calculated flow. Finally, because flow is usually measured per kilogram of estimated fetal weight, this estimation either determined by palpation, extrapolation from birth weight, or by ultrasonic assessment introduced at best an additional 15% inaccuracy.

FLOW VELOCITY WAVE FORM ANALYSIS

Since both blood flow and velocity measurements were dependent on these factors, it became apparent that with present technology these would not be clinically useful parameters to follow. Recognizing these limitations, Schulman et al.[9] studied not blood flow or blood velocity but the FVWFs themselves. The FVWFs are independent of the angle of insonation, vessel diameter, or estimated fetal weight, and these parameters no longer needed to be determined. The measured Doppler shifts were a reflection of the pulsatility (i.e., systolic flow) and downstream vessel resistance (i.e., diastolic flow). The importance and reproducibility of these measurements have been confirmed by others.[10,11]

Although FVWFs appear initially difficult to interpret to a sonologist accustomed to real-time, two-dimensional visual output, they can be interpreted easily with the use of standard ratios involving systolic and diastolic flow velocities. The three most commonly used ratios are the systolic/diastolic, or A/B, ratio,[12] resistance index,[13] and pulsatility index.[14]

A/B = S/D = Systolic/Diastolic ratio
(A − B)/A = Resistance Index
(A − B)/Mean flow = Pulsatility Index

The pulsatility index has an advantage over the other two ratios in the important situation of low or undetectable diastolic flow. In this case the A/B ratio goes to infinity and becomes undefined when there is no diastolic flow; the resistance index becomes unity; and only the pulsatility index remains meaningful at low diastolic flow. Campbell et al.[15] in 1983 introduced the flow index profile, in which pulsatility index was calculated at 0.04-second intervals and plotted as a percentage of mean flow against time.

The FVWF becomes meaningful once it is clear that each major vessel in the uteroplacental unit has a characteristic wave form. A diagram showing an example of FVWF is shown in Figure 11–2. Examples of actual pictures of FVWFs are shown in Figure 11–3. The umbilical vein FVWF is characterized by nonpulsatile flow in the opposite direction to the characteristic umbilical artery flow. The fetal aortic FVWF is characterized by its sharp peak and fall with systole and very low diastolic flow. The fetal heart pattern reveals marked turbulence with two peaks in each cycle. Of more importance are the FVWFs of the vessels feeding both sides of the placenta, the umbilical artery, and the arcuate branches of the uterine vessels. In the normal state both vessels have high flow throughout diastole; indeed, both diastolic flows increase with gestational age. Therefore the S/D ratio in normal pregnancies in the umbilical artery declines from 2.8 to 2.2 from 25 weeks to term.[9]

High diastolic flows imply a low-resistance capillary network, which is necessary for appropriate transplacental exchange. Maternal uterine artery blood flow can be similarly recognized by its characteristic FVWF and its slower pulse. In normal pregnancies the uterine artery mean S/D ratio falls in the third trimester, from 1.6 to 1.4.[11] Again, high diastolic flow implies flow into the low-resistance intervillous spaces. Low resistance is necessary to promote appropriate gas and nutrient exchange.

FLOW VELOCITY WAVE FORM AND IUGR

Once normal FVWF patterns were recognized, Doppler studies were performed in patients at risk for obstetric problems, especially intrauterine growth retardation (IUGR). Table 11–1 summarizes the results in several recently published series for the detection of IUGR.

The simplest technique used in these studies was the blind continuous-wave technique.[18] Vessels were recognized by their audio characteristics and wave form. Criticisms of this technique were described earlier. The continuous-wave directed systems overcame these criticisms because the vessel was visualized in real time and the continuous-wave Doppler was guided into

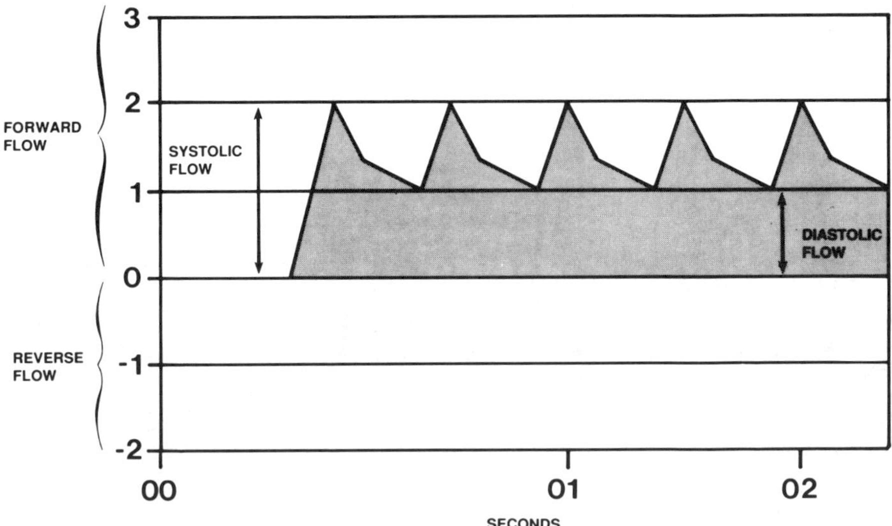

FIG 11–2.
Diagram of a typical umbilical artery flow velocity wave form. All flow is forward in systole and diastole, and this implies low (normal) downstream impedance.

place after the real-time scanner was removed. The pulsed-wave duplex gated systems remain the most precise for blood flow measurements. These systems have not been available for clinical use in the United States because their intensities exceed U.S. Food and Drug Administration regulations limiting fetal exposure to ultrasonic intensity of less than 100 mW/cm^2. Until lower intensity duplex scanners can be developed, studies in the United States will continue to be performed with either blind or directed continuous-wave systems.

It is of note that the studies listed in Table 11–1 can be divided into those in which flow profiles are studied on the fetal side in the fetal aorta or umbilical artery or on the maternal side in the uterine artery. Decrease or loss of diastolic flow on either side of the placenta has been demonstrated to be of considerable concern. Failure of the arcuate vessels to demonstrate high diastolic flow would imply failure to develop appropriate maternal perfusion to the placenta and very high risk for IUGR. Examples of FVWFs with normal and abnormal flow in a fetal umbilical artery are shown in Figure 11–4. The umbilical arteries from a normal twin and a severely growth-retarded twin are shown in Figure 11–5. It is hypothesized that this is caused by a failure of trophoblastic invasion and subsequent failure to induce high arcuate flows.

Campbell[21] has begun to use uterine artery flow studies in the second trimester as an early screening test for high-risk pregnancies. Recent studies have examined term and preterm growth-retarded fetuses separately.[22, 23]

Demonstration of poor diastolic flow in the arcuate branches of the uterine artery as early as 18 weeks' gestation has been shown to be associated with a high incidence of growth-retarded and compromised fetuses in the third trimester.

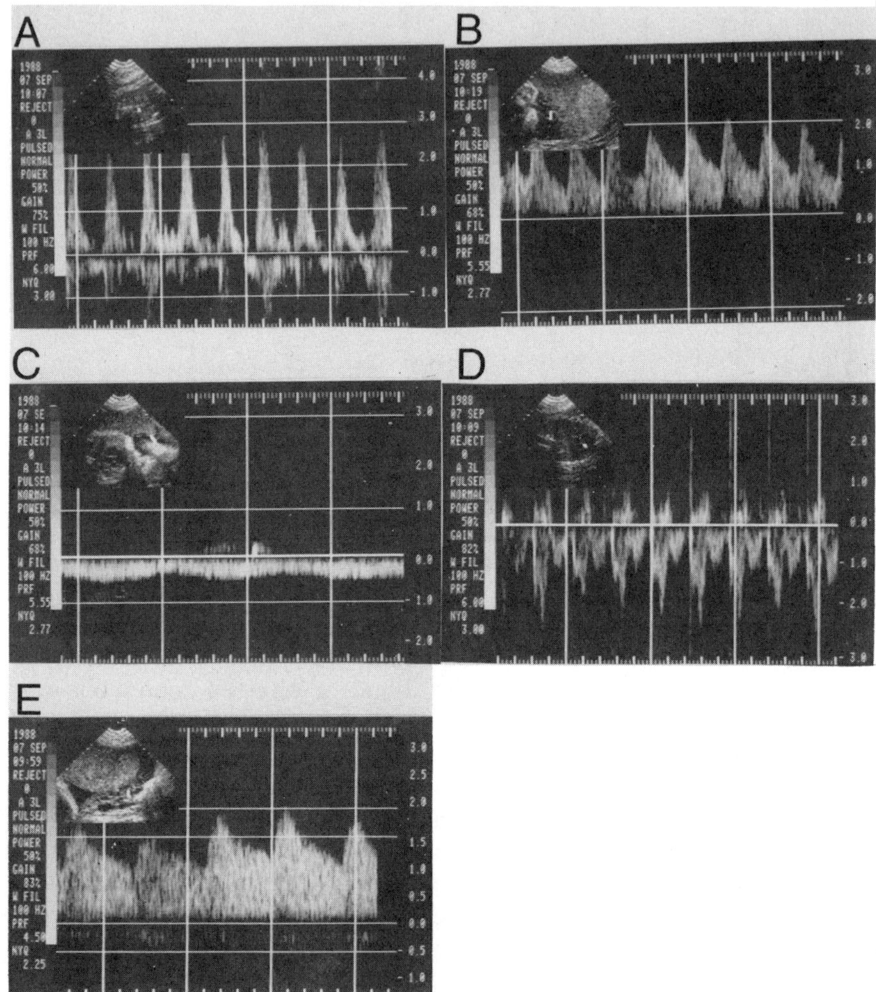

FIG 11–3.

The flow velocity wave form has a characteristic appearance for each vessel as shown. A, fetal aorta has a high systolic flow with no diastolic component. B, the positive channel shows a characteristic wave form for an umbilical artery. C, the negative channel shows the umbilical vein with flow in the opposite direction as the umbilical artery shown in B. D, the fetal heart has a characteristic biphasic and double-peaked pattern. E, the maternal arcuate artery.

TABLE 11–1.
Review of Published Studies for Detection of IUGR by Doppler Flow Studies*

		Vessel	IUGR/Total Patients	Sensitivity (%)
Griffin et al.[10]	PW Duplex	F.T.A.	20/118	75
Trudinger et al.[16]	CW Directed	U.A.	43/136	74
Trudinger et al.[17]	CW Directed	U.A.	25/91	60
Fleischer et al.[18]	CW Blind	U.A.	23/137	78
Trudinger et al.[19]	CW Directed	U.A.	47/164	66
Erskine and Ritchie[20]	PW Duplex	U.A.	9/24	100
			167/670	

n = 427 Sensitivity 64% Specificity 86%
Positive predictive value 67.7%
Negative predictive value 84%

*CW = continuous wave; PW = pulsed wave; FTA = fetal thoracic aorta; UA = umbilical artery.

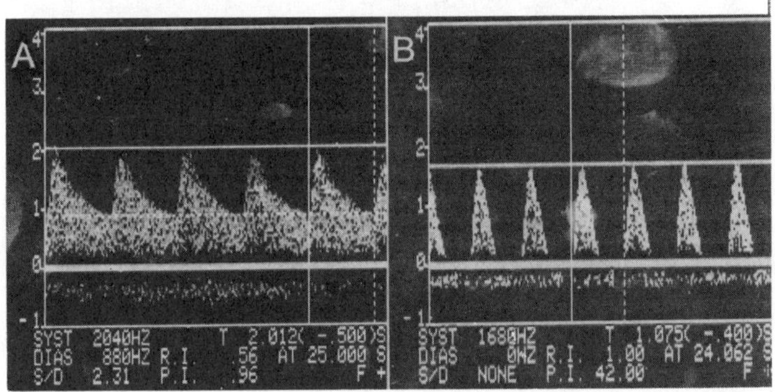

FIG 11–4.
A, example of a flow velocity wave form from a normal umbilical artery. Systolic/diastolic ratio (*S/D*) is normal. **B**, example of a flow velocity wave form from an umbilical artery with minimal diastolic flow. S/D is markedly abnormal.

PATHOPHYSIOLOGIC CORRELATION

Loss of diastolic flow in the umbilical artery or fetal aorta implies similar high risk. This has been shown by Giles et al.[24] to be caused by a failure of development or subsequent obliteration of the tertiary villi. In pregnancies with normal diastolic flow, seven to eight small arteries <90 μm in diameter were found per microscopic field. These small arteries create the low-resistance network necessary to promote high diastolic flow. In those pregnancies with poor diastolic flow, only one to two arteries were found. This finding enhances the pathophysiologic basis for blood flow studies and improves our understanding of the causes of IUGR and of perinatal asphyxia.

FLOW VOLUME WAVE FORM AND FETAL COMPROMISE

Loss of diastolic flow on either side of the placenta places the pregnancy at risk. In several of the studies in Table 11–1, if IUGR did not occur in pregnancies with low diastolic flow, then frequently there were other perinatal problems, such as low Apgar scores, preeclampsia, pregnancy-induced hypertension, or diabetes. Trudinger et al.[19] recognized this and have recently reported a comparison of umbilical artery wave form analysis with nonstress tests to determine fetal compromise. They reported a 3.5-fold improvement in sensitivity for detecting the fetus with IUGR or low Apgar scores when using blood flow studies, as compared with nonstress tests. The specificity and the true positive and negative rates were similar.[19] Blood flow studies

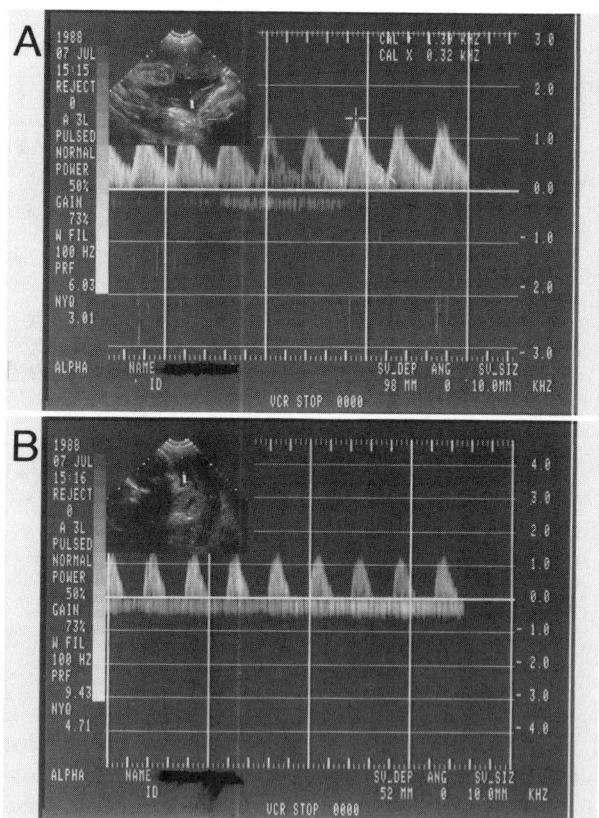

FIG 11–5.

A Doppler study from the umbilical arteries of a set of discordant twins. **A**, the flow velocity wave form from the umbilical artery in the normally growing twin has a normal S/D. **B**, the flow velocity wave form from the severely growth retarded twin (absense of diastolic flow).

are also quicker to perform than nonstress tests or biophysical profiles and are not dependent on fetal activity, fetal sleep cycles, or visualizing of fetal breathing movements. There is as yet not enough data comparing the nonstress test and FVWF to draw any conclusions regarding their relative clinical efficacy.

Of interest, Campbell,[21] using blood flow studies in fetuses with IUGR, has been able to differentiate those fetuses who are healthy but constitutionally small from those who are small and compromised by the presence or absence of diastolic flow.

SUMMARY

Doppler ultrasound is a new method of studying the fetus. Loss of diastolic flow on either side of the placenta may be associated with a hostile intrauterine environment and result in either growth retardation or other poor perinatal outcome. The pathophysiologic basis for these findings has been postulated, but precisely how these studies will be used clinically remains to be seen.[23, 24] They may be used as a screening tool in the second trimester to isolate pregnancies at risk. They may be used in the third trimester to corroborate real-time imaging or as part of antenatal surveillance. Recent studies have found that fetal blood flow measurements can accurately detect discordant growth in twins.[25] At our perinatal center we are currently using umbilical artery blood flow studies on a trial basis after equivocal or nonreactive nonstress tests and in patients with hypertensive complications in pregnancy. Although we are currently not using this information clinically, we have been impressed with the correlation of fetal compromise with poor diastolic flow. Similarly, we have noted good outcomes, Apgar scores, and toleration of labor in fetuses with normal diastolic flow. Just as in the past ten years most biochemical studies for fetal well-being have been replaced by biophysical ultrasound evaluations, the next ten years may find nonstress tests and oxytocin challenge tests yielding to Doppler blood flow studies.

REFERENCES

1. Fitzgerald DE, Drumm JE: Non-invasive measurements of fetal circulation using ultrasound: A new method. *Br Med J* 1977; 2:1450.
2. McCallum WD, Williams CS, Napel S, et al: Fetal blood velocity waveforms. *Am J Obstet Gynecol* 1978; 132:425.
3. Eik-Nes SH, Brubakk AO, Ulstein MK: Measurement of human fetal blood flow. *Lancet* 1980; 1:283.
4. Griffin D, Bilardo K, Diaz J, et al: The measurement of human fetal blood flow with linear array pulsed Doppler duplex scanner. *Eur J Obstet Gynecol Reprod Biol* 1983; 15:462.

5. Griffin D, Cohen-Overbeek T, Campbell S: Fetal and utero-placental blood flow. *Clin Obstet Gynaecol* 1983; 10:565.
6. Gill RW, Trudinger BJ, Garrett WJ, et al: Fetal umbilical venous flow measured in utero by pulsed Doppler and B mode ultrasound. *Am J Obstet Gynecol* 1981; 139:720.
7. Van Lierde M, Oberweis D, Thomas K: Ultrasonic measurement of aortic and umbilical blood flow in the human fetus. *Obstet Gynecol* 1984; 63:801.
8. Erskine RLA, Ritchie JWK: Quantitative measurement of fetal blood flow using Doppler ultrasound. *Br J Obstet Gynaecol* 1985; 92:600.
9. Schulman H, Fleischer A, Stern W, et al: Umbilical velocity wave ratios in human pregnancy. *Am J Obstet Gynecol* 1984; 148:985.
10. Griffin D, Bilardo K, Masini L, et al: Doppler blood flow wave forms in the descending thoracic aorta of the human fetus. *Br J Obstet Gynaecol* 1984; 91:997.
11. Trudinger BJ, Giles WB, Cook CM: Flow velocity wave forms in the maternal uteroplacental and fetal umbilical placental circulations. *Am J Obstet Gynecol* 1985; 152:155.
12. Stuart B, Drumm J, Fitzgerald DE, et al: Fetal blood velocity wave forms in normal pregnancy. *Br J Obstet Gynaecol* 1980; 87:780.
13. Porcelot L: Applicaions cliniques de l'examen Doppler trancutanie, in Peronneau P (ed): *Velocimetric Ultrasonor Doppler*. Inserm October 7-11. 1974; 34:625.
14. Gosling RG, King DH: Ultrasound angiology, in Marcus AN, Adamson L (eds): *Arteries and Veins*. New York, Churchill Livingstone, 1975, pp 61-98.
15. Campbell S, Griffin DR, Pearce JM, et al: New Doppler technique for assessing uteroplacental blood flow. *Lancet* 1983; 1:675.
16. Trudinger BJ, Giles WB, Cook CM: Fetal umbilical artery velocity wave forms and placental resistance: Clinical significance. *Br J Obstet Gynaecol* 1985; 92:23.
17. Trudinger BJ, Giles WB, Cook CM: Uteroplacental blood flow velocity-time wave forms in normal and complicated pregnancy. *Br J Obstet Gynaecol* 1985; 92:39.
18. Fleischer A, Schulman H, Farmakides G, et al: Umbilical artery velocity waveforms and intrauterine growth retardation. *Am J Obstet Gynecol* 1985; 151:502.
19. Trudinger BJ, Cook CM, Jones L, et al: A comparison of fetal heart ratio monitoring and umbilical artery wave forms in the recognition of fetal compromise. *Br J Obstet Gynaecol* 1986; 93:171.
20. Erskine RLA, Ritchie JWK: Umbilical artery blood flow characteristics in normal and growth retarded fetuses. *Br J Obstet Gynaecol* 1985; 92:605.
21. Campbell S: Fetal Blood Flow Studies International Symposium on Perinatal Ultrasound, Norfolk, VA, March 1986.
22. McCowan LM, Erskine LA, Ritchie K: Umbilical artery doppler blood flow studies in the preterm small for gestational age fetus. *Am J Obstet Gynecol* 1987; 156:655.
23. Fleischer A, Anyaegbunam AA, Schulman H, et al: Uterine and umbilical artery velocimetry during normal labor. *Am J Obstet Gynecol* 1987; 157:40.
24. Giles WB, Trudinger BJ, Baird PJ: Fetal umbilical artery flow velocity waveforms and placental resistance: Pathological correlation. *Br J Obstet Gynaecol* 1985; 92:31.

25. Gerson AG, Wallace DM, Bridgens NK: Duplex Doppler ultrasound in the evaluation of growth in twin pregnancies. *Obstet Gynecol* 1987; 70:419.

PART V

Management

12

Management of Intrauterine Growth Retardation

Robert Resnik, M.D.

Once the diagnosis of fetal intrauterine growth retardation (IUGR) has been confirmed, the clinician assumes several responsibilities with regard to management, including appropriate counseling of the prospective parents, a diligent search for the cause of aberrant growth, continuing antepartum evaluation of fetal growth and well-being, correct timing of delivery, meticulous intrapartum monitoring, and neonatal consultation. The purpose of this chapter is to explore these individual requirements and to define the rationale for current management approaches.

PARENTAL COUNSELING

Frequently the pregnant patient is aware that fetal growth has been suboptimal and brings this observation to the attention of her obstetrician. Even among primigravid women who may be uncertain as to what represents an appropriate size for gestational age, friends or family will rarely hesitate to point out discrepancies. Indeed, the first suspicion of IUGR may be the result of a patient's voiced concerns. After the diagnosis is confirmed, appropriate counseling must be provided to the parents. Clinicians should provide emotional support with a reasonably optimistic yet realistic approach to outcome as it relates to antepartum findings. For example, IUGR noted before 26 weeks, particularly when associated with oligohydramnios, has an almost uniformly poor outcome. Conversely, abnormal fetal growth occurring later, particularly when due to primary placental dysfunction or preeclampsia, is usually associated with a favorable outcome provided appropriate perinatal management is provided.

With prospective parents it is useful to use such terms as "slow fetal growth" or "small for gestational age" rather than "intrauterine growth retardation." When the common medical terminology is used parents tend to hear only the word "retardation," which may not accurately reflect long-term prognosis.

SEARCH FOR CAUSE

The causes of IUGR are multifactorial and may be difficult to identify in any individual patient. Nevertheless, it is important to determine the cause, if possible, because management and prognosis will be influenced by knowledge of the underlying disorder.

Perhaps the most common identifiable cause of IUGR is maternal vascular disease. Long-standing preeclampsia or chronic hypertensive disease with superimposed preeclampsia may decrease intervillous blood flow[1] and produce placental infarcts that decrease trophoblastic surface area for nutrient transport and respiratory gas exchange. Maternal vascular disease due to diabetes mellitus may also result in IUGR. Finally, women who have a circulating lupus anticoagulant with or without other criteria for clinical lupus erythematosus frequently have growth-retarded fetuses.[2] Preeclampsia and lupus anticoagulant are characterized by a specific decidual vascular lesion, atherosis, which decreases the lumen of spiral arterioles and uterine blood flow.[2,3] It is worth emphasizing that preeclampsia is a multiorgan disease and may have a negative influence on fetal growth well before clinical evidence of maternal hypertension or proteinuria.

Fetal infections, particularly early in pregnancy, may deleteriously affect fetal growth. Rubella, although no longer a significant health problem, is known to influence cell growth during organogenesis.[4] However, cytomegalovirus is prevalent in the general population and is known to be cytotoxic to the developing fetus, resulting in lower than normal organ weights.[5] Congenital syphilis and toxoplasmosis occur far less frequently than other infectious vectors in terms of their impact on fetal growth. A careful history to detect possible infection and appropriate use of acute and convalescent antibody titers from maternal blood will be helpful in detecting an infectious origin of IUGR.

Chromosomal abnormalities and other congenital malformations are frequently associated with poor fetal growth. For example, infants with trisomies 21, 18, or 13 are often small for gestational age.[6] Malformations of multifactorial origin also may be associated with poor prenatal growth as part of a larger syndrome. A thorough ultrasound evaluation of fetal anatomy is indicated after the diagnosis of IUGR, and amniocentesis for chromosome analysis may be considered under special circumstances.

Multiple gestations are responsible for approximately 10% of intrauterine growth retarded infants, and it has long been known that the rate of fetal growth decreases among twins and triplets compared with singletons after 26 to 28 weeks gestation.[7] Again ultrasound studies will confirm the presence of a multiple gestation, but special attention should be directed toward signs of placental vascular communication such as markedly discordant growth, hydramnios, or the inability to identify a membrane separating the fetuses.

Other identifiable causes of poor fetal growth include life-style in which there is excessive use of alcohol or tobacco and prescribed drugs such as the hydantoin derivatives and warfarin. Poor maternal nutrition rarely produces significant fetal growth retardation.

Utilizing a combination of appropriate laboratory testing together with a careful history, it is possible to identify a cause for fetal growth retardation in as many as half of cases before delivery.

ANTEPARTUM SURVEILLANCE

It is well known that the perinatal mortality rate among intrauterine growth-retarded fetuses and infants is much higher than that for their appropriately grown counterparts. Scott and Usher[8] reported 20 years ago that the stillbirth rate was eight times higher for infants below the 2.5th percentile of birth weight for gestational age. More recently Williams et al.[9] reported that neonates weighing between 1,500 and 2,500 gm at 38 to 42 weeks gestation had a perinatal mortality rate between 5 and 30 times that of normally grown infants. From this information it is logical to conclude that close attention to fetal growth and oxygenation is imperative. Antepartum evaluation includes the use of ultrasound and fetal heart rate testing. Although endocrine tests no longer have a significant role in fetal evaluation, maternal serum estriol and human placental lactogen (HPL) testing are briefly reviewed.

Estriol and Human Placental Lactogen

The morphologic and biochemical aberrations of IUGR theoretically lend themselves ideally to management by serial estriol determination. Most studies demonstrate low to low normal estriol concentrations in maternal urine or serum. This may be due to atrophy of the fetal adrenal zone in intrauterine growth-retarded neonates[10] or to a decrease in the availability of the estriol precursor dehydroepiandrosterone sulfate.[11] The main problem in clinical usage is due in part to the overlap between low and normal values and to the difficulty in distinguishing what represents a significant decrease from an already low concentration. Whereas estriol values may be of help if they are well into the normal range or if they are rising, a low to low normal value will not assist in management.

The same problems apply to the use of HPL as a guide to management. Although the concentration of HPL in maternal plasma is low (less than 4 μg/ml) in the majority of intrauterine growth-retarded pregnancies after week 36 of gestation, there is a great deal of overlap between normal and abnormal values.

Ultrasound

The use of high-resolution modern ultrasound equipment currently is the cornerstone of diagnosis of abnormal fetal growth and its serial evaluation. The first step is a thorough examination of the fetal anatomy with special attention to the central nervous system, urinary tract, cardiovasculature, and limb length. Within the limits of current ultrasound technology, the majority of major congenital malformations can be detected with accuracy.

Attention is then turned to an estimate of fetal weight. Several studies have demonstrated the accuracy of computer-derived formulas in estimating fetal weight and its application to low birth weight or growth-retarded fetus.[12–15]

At our institution estimated fetal weight is derived from measurements of fetal head and abdominal circumference and femur length (Fig 12–1).[15] Initial and serial measurement of these dimensions allow for the accurate diagnosis of IUGR and enable the clinician to determine the rate of growth with advancing gestation. Finally, the comparison of measurements that are dependent on skeletal development, in contrast to those influenced by organ size and depth of subcutaneous tissue, enables the clinician to determine the pattern of growth abnormalities, namely, where on the spectrum between asymmetric and symmetric growth retardation an individual fetus lies. It should be emphasized that accurate knowledge of gestational age is required, because all measurements are evaluated based on this variable.

That IUGR is often associated with oligohydramnios can also be used by the clinician to aid in the diagnosis. During the latter half of pregnancy the majority of amnionic fluid is derived from fetal urination, and urinary production rates are generally lower in the growth-retarded fetus,[16] presumably as a consequence of decreased fetal plasma volume and renal blood flow. This has clinical relevance with respect to diagnosis, because the ultrasonic observation of oligohydramnios alone should raise suspicion of IUGR. In one study of 31 fetuses noted to be growth retarded at birth, 83% demonstrated decreased amnionic fluid volume antepartum.[17]

Studies are under way to see if IUGR can be predicted from evaluation of the waveforms of the umbilical artery.[18] In addition, the technology is now available to study blood flow in the uterine artery.[19] The use of ultrasound and doppler blood flow measurements to diagnose IUGR are described in detail in Chapters 10 and 11.

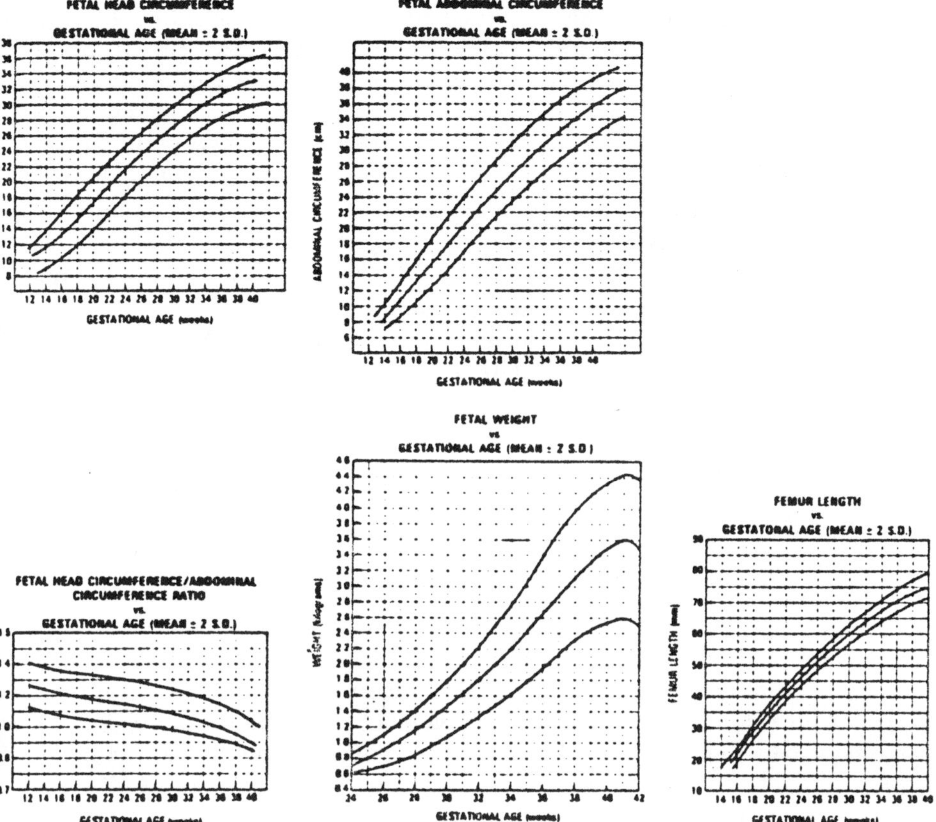

FIG 12–1.
Composite of fetal body measurements used for studies of fetal growth. (From Creasy RK, Resnik R: Intrauterine growth retardation, in Creasy RK, Resnik R (eds): *Maternal-Fetal Medicine: Principles and Practice*. Philadelphia, WB Saunders Co, 1984. Used by permission.)

Antepartum Fetal Function Tests

Testing to determine fetal well-being should be initiated shortly after diagnosis and counseling are completed. There is considerable debate as to which among the nonstress test, contraction stress test, or biophysical profile is the appropriate method to evaluate fetal health for any high-risk pregnancy condition, including IUGR. It is not the purpose of this chapter to delve into the relative merits of the various tests. However, given the high-risk nature of IUGR with its high frequency of fetal death and hypoxia during labor, a few points deserve emphasis.

Abundant evidence has been obtained from clinical studies and basic laboratory investigation using animal models that, with respect to fetal heart rate as an indicator of fetal health, late decelerations precede the loss of baseline heart rate variability and accelerations. Following this logic, it is reasonable to conclude that a contraction stress test (oxytocin or nipple stimulation induced) would be an earlier and more sensitive indicator of fetal hypoxia and therefore a more appropriate test. Indeed, a positive contraction stress test is frequently observed with the intrauterine growth-retarded fetus.[20] Although the nonstress test alone may be an adequate screening device for many high-risk pregnancies, its predictive accuracy is surely enhanced by use of other components of the biophysical profile, which include the delineation and scoring of amnionic fluid volume and fetal tone, movement, and respiratory activity.[21] A negative contraction stress test or a high biophysical profile score is reassuring, but should be repeated at 1- to 3-day intervals in the growth-retarded fetus.

TIME OF DELIVERY

Opinions are divided with respect to when the fetus with IUGR should be delivered. One school of thought favors delivery when fetal growth curves demonstrate poor or absent growth, suggesting that the intrauterine environment is no longer suited to fetal health. Conversely, others point out that a slow rate of fetal growth is a compensatory mechanism to maintain survival and that there is no data base to support preterm delivery. In fact, this issue cannot be resolved based on current evidence. Most authorities agree that the fetus with absence of fetal growth over a time period as a consequence of maternal hypertensive disease should be delivered early regardless of the degree of lung maturity. However, because preterm delivery may result in respiratory distress syndrome and other complications of prematurity,[22] and because amnionic fluid analysis of phospholipids for lung maturity may not be possible, the importance of careful antepartum heart rate testing is reemphasized when aberrant growth due to other causes has been determined. Clearly, nonreassuring fetal function tests warrant delivery regardless of gestational age and the state of fetal lung maturity.

INTRAPARTUM MONITORING

It has long been recognized that IUGR is associated with a higher rate of intrapartum stillbirth, low Apgar score, and meconium aspiration. In one study almost half of the growth-retarded infants had moderate to severe metabolic acidosis at delivery, as determined by a reduction in the umbilical artery buffer base.[23] These findings document the importance of fetal heart rate monitoring and scalp blood pH testing during labor. Cesarean section should be seriously considered when delivery is indicated in the absence of an inducible cervix or with early signs of fetal distress during labor.

NEONATAL CONSULTATION

The constellation of neonatal problems associated with IUGR is discussed elsewhere in this text. It is clear that the neonatologist will be treating an infant who may have birth asphyxia and its complications, or metabolic problems such as hypoglycemia, hypocalcemia, and polycythemia. In addition, infections may present risks to other infants in the nursery and to nursing personnel. Finally, the skills of a pediatric dysmorphologist, pediatric surgeon, or geneticist may be required. For these reasons the pediatrician should be involved shortly after the diagnosis of IUGR is made in order that any necessary special arrangements can be made before delivery and for continuity of parental counseling.

In summary, after diagnosis of IUGR in a pregnancy, a specific plan of management is indicated incorporating the major issues discussed in this text.

REFERENCES

1. Browne JCM, Veall N: The maternal placental blood flow in normotensive and hypertensive woman. *J Obstet Gynaecol Br Commonw* 1953; 60:141.
2. Lubbe WF, Butler WS, Palmer SJ, et al: Lupus anticoagulant in pregnancy. *Br J Obstet Gynaecol* 1984; 91:357.
3. Brosens IA, Robertson WB, Dickson HG: The role of the spiral arteries in the pathogenesis of preeclampsia. *Obstet Gynecol Annu* 1972; 1:171.
4. Alford CA Jr: Rubella, in Remington JS, Kline JO (eds): *Infectious Diseases of the Fetus and Newborn Infant.* Philadelphia, WB Saunders Co, 1976.
5. Kline JO, Remington JS, Marcy SM: Current concepts of infections of the fetus and newborn infant, in Remington JS, Kline JO (eds): *Infectious Diseases of the Fetus and Newborn Infant*, ed 2. Philadelphia, WB Saunders Co, 1983.
6. Chen ATL, Chan Y-K, Falek A: The effects of chromosome abnormalities on birth weight and man. II: Autosomal defect. *Hum Hered* 1972; 22:209.
7. McKeown T, Record RG: Observations on fetal growth and multiple pregnancy in man. *J Endocrinol* 1952; 8:386.
8. Scott KE, Usher R: Fetal malnutrition: Its incidence, causes and effects. *Am J Obstet Gynecol* 1966; 94:951.
9. Williams RL, Creasy RK, Cunningham GC, et al: Fetal growth and perinatal viability in California. *Obstet Gynecol* 1982; 59:624.
10. Naeye RL: Malnutrition: Probable causes of fetal growth retardation. *Arch Pathol* 1965; 79:284.
11. Turnipseed MR, Bentley K, Reynolds JW: Serum dehydroepiandrosterone sulfate in premature infants and infants with intrauterine growth retardation. *J Clin Endocrinol Metab* 1976; 43:1219.
12. Shepard MT, Richards VM, Berkowitz RT, et al: An evaluation of two equations for the prediction of fetal weight by ultrasound. *Am J Obstet Gynecol* 1982; 136:45.
13. Crane JP, Kopta MM: Prediction of intrauterine growth retardation via ultraso-

nically measured of head/abdominal circumference ratios. *Obstet Gynecol* 1979; 54:597.

14. Ott WJ, Doyle S: Ultrasonic diagnosis of altered fetal growth by use of a normal ultrasonic fetal weight curve. *Obstet Gynecol* 1984; 63:201.
15. Creasy RK, Resnik R: Intrauterine growth retardation, in Creasy RK, Resnik R (eds): *Maternal-Fetal Medicine: Principles and Practice.* Philadelphia, WB Saunders Co, 1984.
16. Kurjak A, Kirkinen P, Latin V, et al: Ultrasonic assessment of fetal kidney function in normal and complicated pregnancies. *Am J Obstet Gynecol* 1981; 141:266.
17. Manning FA, Hill LM, Platt LD: Qualitative amnionic fluid volume determination by ultrasound: Antepartum detection of intrauterine growth retardation. *Am J Obstet Gynecol* 1981; 139:254.
18. McCowan LM, Erskine LA, Ritchie K: Umbilical artery doppler blood flow studies in the preterm small for gestational age fetus. *Am J Obstet Gynecol* 1987; 156:655.
19. Fleischer A, Anyaegbunam AA, Schulman H, et al: Uterine and umbilical artery velocimetry during normal labor. *Am J Obstet Gynecol* 1987; 157:40.
20. Cetrulo CL, Freeman RF: Bioelectric evaluation in intrauterine growth retardation. *Clin Obstet Gynecol* 1977; 20:979.
21. Manning FA, Lange IR, Morrison I, et al: Fetal biophysical profiles score and the non-stress test: A comparative trial. *Obstet Gynecol* 1984; 64:326.
22. Perry CP, Harris RE, DeLemos RA, et al: IUGR infants: Correlation of gestational with maternal factors, mode of delivery and perinatal survival. *Obstet Gynecol* 1976; 48:182.
23. Low JA, Boston RW, Pancham SR: Fetal asphyxia during the antepartum period in intrauterine growth retarded infants. *Am J Obstet Gynecol* 1972; 113:351.

13

Antepartum Fetal Monitoring in the Growth-Retarded Fetus

Thomas L. Gross, M.D.

Antepartum tests of fetal well-being have become standard in managing pregnancies at risk. Frequent assessment of fetal health is especially important when the fetus is suspected to be growth retarded. The goal in assessing the fetus in these pregnancies is to detect chronic hypoxia with its potential morbidity and to prevent intrauterine fetal death.

The antepartum tests of fetal welfare used commonly over the last 15 years can be divided into three groups: biochemical studies of maternal blood, electronic fetal heart rate monitoring, and biophysical parameters related to amniotic fluid volume, fetal muscle tone, and movement. Biochemical studies of maternal blood (i.e., estriol and human placental lactogen) are no longer used. However, both antepartum fetal heart rate testing and the biophysical profile (BPP) have their proponents, and at present there is not uniform agreement as to which is most applicable in the at-risk fetus. This chapter outlines how these tests are used and some of their advantages and disadvantages.

Various aspects of antepartum testing must be evaluated when recommending which tests are most appropriate. First, the accuracy of a test in predicting an abnormal outcome (i.e., frequency of false negative results) must be evaluated. That is, how often is a normal test followed by an abnormal outcome, such as delivery of a depressed neonate or intrauterine fetal death. A second important aspect is how often a positive test result suggesting fetal distress is actually followed by delivery of a healthy neonate (i.e., false positive rate). One possible morbidity related to a test with a high false positive rate is that a group of fetuses may be delivered at an unnecessarily premature gestation. Finally, the question of which tests are most readily available in all hospitals so that they can be widely applied in the entire population must also be taken into account.

ANTEPARTUM FETAL HEART RATE MONITORING

Nonstress Test

At present the simplest and most widely available antepartum test is the nonstress test (NST). The electronic fetal monitor is used to measure accelerations of the fetal heart rate that occur with fetal movement. A normal or reactive test is defined as one in which at least two fetal heart rate accelerations (of at least 15 beats per minute) occur over 20 minutes. A reactive NST suggests that the fetal central nervous system is intact and well oxygenated. In a nonreactive NST fetal heart rate accelerations above the baseline do not occur or are less than 15 beats per minute. If the test is nonreactive, the 20-minute period normally used must be extended for at least an additional 40 minutes, and several investigators have suggested that the test must be extended for at least 120 minutes. Other indications of possible fetal distress on an NST are a baseline fetal heart rate of less than 120 or more than 160 beats per minute, spontaneous decelerations, or decelerations in association with spontaneous uterine contractions.

Contraction Stress Test

The contraction stress test (CST) is performed by administering low-dose intravenous oxytocin by infusion pump to stimulate three uterine contractions in ten minutes. Recurrent late decelerations are often associated with fetal compromise. The mother must not be tested lying flat on her back, but tilted to one side, because the supine position can decrease uterine blood flow and cause late decelerations in a normal fetus.

An alternate method for inducing contractions that is increasing in popularity is the nipple stimulation test. Stimulation of maternal breasts results in the release of endogenous oxytocin, which produces uterine contractions. Both maternal nipple stimulation and intravenous infusion of oxytocin can result in uterine hypertonus that can cause the normal fetus to have late decelerations. The nipple stimulation test must be performed with caution, with stimulation of only one maternal nipple to lessen the chance of uterine hypertonus.

PREDICTIVE VALUE OF ANTEPARTUM FETAL HEART RATE MONITORING

There are no large series examining antepartum monitoring that include only pregnancies with growth-retarded fetuses. The results of a prospective multi-institutional study of more than 18,000 antepartum tests in nearly 7,500 high-risk patients in which antepartum fetal heart rate testing was evaluated are helpful because more than 11% of the patients were studied because of intrauterine growth retardation (IUGR).[1] After correcting for fatal congenital anomalies, there were three antepartum fetal deaths within a week of a reactive NST (1.4 in 1,000),[1] and no antepartum deaths within a week of a negative CST.

As can be seen in Table 13–1, nonreactive NSTs and positive CSTs are associated with increased fetal morbidity. However, the most common outcome was a 5-minute Apgar score >7.[1] These high false positive rates with antepartum fetal heart rate tests remain a problem and raise the potential for unnecessary intervention. In a collaborative study of 7,500 pregnancies, 16 mothers were delivered because of abnormal fetal heart rate, with subsequent neonatal respiratory distress syndrome (RDS), although none of the cases resulted in perinatal deaths. This suggests that in this study carried out in large university centers the potential for unnecessary intervention resulting in RDS was present but was rare, and neonatal death due to unnecessary intervention did not occur at all. This excellent outcome in spite of the very high false positive rate is likely due to the great deal of experience of the physicians in the centers participating in the study. Antepartum fetal heart rate testing has been available for more than a decade, and physicians have learned how to use it.

COMBINED NONSTRESS TEST AND CONTRACTION STRESS TEST

The rare occurrence of fetal loss when using antepartum fetal heart rate testing as a sole means to monitor fetal well-being points out that both the NST and CST are valuable. However, some intrauterine deaths still occur after a reactive NST, so this method cannot be used alone in very high-risk patients, including those with a growth-retarded fetus. A protocol for using the NST and CST in combination is shown in Table 13–2. The baseline fetal heart rate is evaluated as either reactive or nonreactive; then a CST is performed and the results recorded as negative or positive. The combined test results are then classified as reactive-negative CST, nonreactive-negative CST, reactive-positive CST, or nonreactive-positive CST. The false negative rate with this combined approach is probably the lowest of any antepartum fetal monitoring test, including the BPP.

TABLE 13–1.
Perinatal Morbidity by Worst Test Result*

Result	IUGR (%)	5-min Apgar Score <7 (%)	Late Deceleration (%)	Fetal Distress (%)
Negative CST	6.8	2.4	8.1	20.2
Reactive NST	6.8	3.4	6.4	19.9
Nonreactive NST	11.4	13.0	12.5	26.3
Reactive Positive CST	27.7	4.4	47.3	62.4
Nonreactive Positive CST	23.9	29.4	71.9	78.1

*Adapted from Freeman RK, et al: *Am J Obstet Gynecol* 1982; 143:771.

This combined approach has a major drawback in that the CST requires the placement of an intravenous line in the patient, which is time consuming and may not be well accepted.

An important point to be remembered when evaluating the fetus with IUGR is the high incidence of congenital abnormalities in this group. It is now well known that one third of all fetal anomalies incompatible with life are associated with abnormal fetal heart rate.[1] This raises the concern for the potential unnecessary intervention in fetuses with fatal anomalies if fetal heart rate testing is used alone to monitor high-risk pregnancies. Because many of these anomalies can be diagnosed by level II ultrasonography, this must be considered when using antepartum fetal heart rate testing.

The growth-retarded fetus is more likely to have oligohydramnios, and the relationship between decreased amniotic fluid and fetal heart rate deceleration, both spontaneous and in association with contractions, is well known. In the patient who is not in labor, these decelerations may not be a sign of fetal distress, and this must be considered when using the NST and CST to evaluate the growth-retarded fetus.

TABLE 13–2.
Protocol for Test Interpretation Using Combined NST and CST*

Reactive: Two or more accelerations exceeding 15 bpm in amplitude and lasting >15 sec during the test.
Nonreactive: Fewer than two accelerations that exceed 15 bpm in amplitude or last >15 sec at any point during the test.
Negative: No late deceleration, with a contraction frequency of at least three in 10 min.
Positive: Consistent and persistent late deceleration, regardless of contraction frequency without excessive uterine activity (hyperstimulation).
Equivocal: Suspicious—nonpersistent late deceleration. Hyperstimulation—fetal heart rate deceleration associated with excessive uterine activity as defined by a contraction frequency of greater than five in 10 min or contraction duration >90 sec.

*Adapted from Freeman RK, et al: *Am J Obstet Gynecol* 1982: 143:771.

FETAL BIOPHYSICAL PARAMETERS

Fetal Breathing Movements

Fetal breathing movements were initially examined as a measure of fetal well-being. Early studies have shown that the fetal animal normally makes breathing movements and that hypoxia is one cause for their cessation. This finding resulted in the suggestion that either a change in the pattern of fetal breathing or its absence could be used as an indicator of fetal distress. This early interest in using fetal breathing alone as a fetal welfare test has now been abandoned because of the many variables that are known to influence fetal respiratory movements in the normal pregnancy. Fetal breathing movements are now included in the BPP.

Biophysical Profile

Manning et al.[2] developed a protocol for assessing fetal well-being that included five fetal biophysical parameters: fetal breathing, gross fetal body movements, fetal muscle tone, amniotic fluid volume, and reactivity of the fetal heart rate (Table 13–3). It was proposed that combining multiple biophysical variables into a profile could improve the ability to predict the fetus destined to die in the perinatal period. The normal appearance of all five of these individual variables is believed to indicate an intact and well-oxygenated fetal central nervous system.

TABLE 13–3.
Technique and Interpretation of Biophysical Profile Scoring*

Biophysical Variable	Normal (score = 2)	Abnormal (score = 0)
Fetal breathing movements	One or more episodes of ≥30 sec in 30 min	Absent or no episode of ≥30 sec in 30 min
Gross body movements	Three or more discrete body/limb movements in 30 min (episodes of active continuous movement considered as single movement)	Two or less episodes of body/limb movements in 30 min
Fetal muscle tone	One or more episodes of active extension with return to flexion of fetal limb(s) or trunk; opening and closing of hand considered normal tone	Either slow extension with return to partial flexion or movement of limb in full extension or absent fetal movement
Reactive fetal heart rate	Two or more episodes of acceleration of ≥15 bpm and of ≥15 sec associated with fetal movement in 20 min	Fewer than two episodes of acceleration of fetal heart rate or acceleration of <15 bpm in 40 min
Qualitative amniotic fluid	One or more pockets of fluid measuring ≥1 cm in two perpendicular planes	Either no pockets or a pocket <1 cm in two perpendicular planes

*Adapted from Manning FA, et al: *Am J Obstet Gynecol* 1987; 156:709.

The fetal BPP has now been modified so that the NST is used only in selected cases in which one or more of the ultrasound parameters is not normal. Used in this way, the false negative rate (fetal death occurring within a week of a normal result) has been reported to be 0.7 in 1,000.[2,3] The scoring of the BPP and its use in pregnancy management are shown in Table 13–4.

Although the BPP does improve the positive predictive value of fetal deaths compared with antepartum fetal heart rate monitoring, the rate of false positive results is still high: 72%.[3] The impact of these false positive results and how often they would be followed by unnecessary intervention, with subsequent neonatal respiratory distress syndrome, has not yet been examined.

The question of which of the five parameters of the BPP are most important in predicting poor outcome has been examined in one study. Baskett et al.[3] found there was no pattern to the predictive value of the individual parameters of the BPP in the eight cases in their study in which perinatal deaths due to asphyxia occurred. Only one of the eight patients had a normal BPP score. Of the predictive ability for perinatal deaths of the single variables, only fetal movement was nearly as accurate as the entire BPP in predicting intrauterine fetal death. However, even fetal movement was abnormal in only four of the eight perinatal deaths. This study suggests that a BPP of several variables is superior to the individual variables, including the antepartum NST, in predicting asphyxia.

There are still several unanswered questions with regard to the BPP.[5] Of major importance is that an abnormal score is thought to be a late sign of fetal hypoxia,[3,5] and in certain cases a positive CST result may actually be an earlier sign of asphyxia.[1] Several aspects of the performance of the BPP are still not standardized. For example, the types of fetal body movement constituting evidence for normal fetal body movement is not agreed on. The assessment of fetal body movement and fetal tone in the patient with severe oligohydramnios (less than 1 cm pocket of amniotic fluid) is impossible using the definitions of some authors for assessing movement and tone. In addition, recent studies have shown that gestational age affects the predictive value of the biophysical parameters.[6] The NST and fetal breathing movements are more likely to be falsely abnormal early in the third trimester, with the other biophysical variables not significantly affected up through 41 weeks.

It now appears clear that a profile of tests is needed to monitor the fetus at severe risk. Which variables will eventually be considered most important is not known at this time.

MONITORING THE FETUS WITH SUSPECTED IUGR

Of the many studies examining antepartum fetal monitoring, the clinician must choose a protocol to observe the growth-retarded fetus. The following

TABLE 13–4.
Biophysical Profile Scoring: Management Protocol*†

Score	Interpretation	Management
10	Normal infant, low risk for chronic asphyxia	Repeat testing at weekly intervals. Repeat testing twice weekly in diabetic patients and pregnancies ≥42 weeks gestation.
8	Normal infant, low risk for chronic asphyxia	Repeat testing at weekly intervals. Repeat testing twice weekly in diabetic patients and pregnancies ≥42 weeks. Oligohydramnios is an indication for delivery.
6	Suspicion of chronic asphyxia	Repeat testing in 4-6 hours. Consider delivery if oligohydramnios is present. Rule out ruptured membranes as a cause of oligohydramnios.
4	Suspicion of chronic asphyxia	If ≥36 weeks and favorable, deliver. If <36 weeks, repeat test in 4-6 hours; if repeat score ≤4, deliver.
0-2	Strong suspicion of chronic asphyxia	Extend testing time to 120 min. If persistent score ≤4, deliver regardless of gestational age.

*Adapted from Manning FA, et al: *Am J Obstet Gynecol* 1981; 140:289.
†Management protocol for use of BPP in entire population of high-risk pregnancies (not limited to intrauterine growth retardation).

protocol takes into account some of the limitations of each technique and tries to place them on a practical level.

Fetal Growth

The fetus with suspected IUGR should be examined with a level II ultrasound study to detect anomalies. Subsequent ultrasound evaluations should be performed every 2 to 3 weeks to monitor serial fetal growth measurements.

Fetal Well-Being/Biophysical Profile

Tests of fetal well-being should be performed one to three times per week, with frequency of monitoring based on the severity of the clinical findings and the time during gestation when the diagnosis is made. The fetal BPP is performed once per week. If more frequent fetal testing is indicated, subsequent fetal welfare studies during the week are performed using the NST. If the fetal heart rate is reactive, the once a week BPP schedule is maintained.

Timing of Delivery

Delivery at ≤34 weeks gestation.—In the patient suspected of having a growth-retarded fetus with a nonreactive NST and a BPP score of 4 or less, management must be individualized. If the test results are equivocal or if the score of 4 on the BPP is based on normal fetal body movements and normal amniotic fluid volume, then temporizing with repeat of the tests in 24 hours may be indicated. Patients with persistent nonreactive NST and a BPP score of 4 or less are candidates for delivery. See Chapter 16, Patient 1, for a more in-depth discussion of timing of delivery in the growth-retarded fetus.

Delivery at >34 weeks gestation.—There is general agreement that in the presence of IUGR and a persistently nonreactive NST and abnormal BPP (score of 4 or less) the fetus should be delivered. Recent studies have suggested delivery if the BPP score is confirmed as 6 or less in the growth-retarded fetus.[2] It is impossible to apply general rules to all pregnancies in patients in which the BPP score is in the range of 4 to 6. Regardless of the gestational age, clinicians with little experience in individualizing the use of the antepartum tests should seek consultation with a physician experienced in dealing with high-risk pregnancy.

Use of amniocentesis.—Prior to delivery in equivocal cases of suspected IUGR, the clinician should consider amniocentesis. One benefit is that the presence of phosphatidylglycerol or a mature L/S ratio in amniotic fluid in a small fetus is strong supportive evidence that IUGR is present.[7] In addition, the presence of phosphatidylglycerol documents final pulmonary maturity and confirms that delivery will not worsen the outcome or cause unnecessary fetal respiratory distress. The oligohydramnios often associated with severe IUGR may make amniocentesis impossible.

Term Gestation.—When to deliver the suspected growth-retarded fetus that is at term gestation or the fetus with documented fetal pulmonary maturity but with normal BPP for fetal well-being is questionable. Some physicians believe that delivery is indicated as soon as pulmonary maturity is documented even though biophysical tests show that fetal well-being is still normal. This approach is based on the assumption that abnormal fetal monitoring test results indicate early signs of asphyxia and that the potentially hostile intrauterine environment may increase the risk of chronic hypoxia and brain damage. Other physicians believe that early delivery by induction of labor will increase fetal distress and result in many cesarean section deliveries that would not have been necessary if labor were awaited. The answer to this question will require future long-term infant follow-up studies.

REFERENCES

1. Freeman RK, Anderson G, Dorchester W: A prospective multi-institutional study of antepartum fetal heart rate monitoring. I: Risk of perinatal mortality and morbidity according to antepartum fetal heart rate test results. *Am J Obstet Gynecol* 1982; 143:771.
2. Manning FA, Morrison I, Lange IR, et al: Fetal biophysical profile scoring: Selective use of the nonstress test. *Am J Obstet Gynecol* 1987; 156:709.
3. Baskett TF, Allen AC, Gray JH, et al: Fetal biophysical profile and perinatal death. *Obstet Gynecol* 1987; 70:357.
4. Manning FA, Baskett TF, Morrison I, et al: Fetal biophysical profile scoring: A prospective study in 1,184 high risk patients. *Am J Obstet Gynecol* 1981; 140:289.
5. Vintzileos AM, Campbell WA, Nochimson DJ, et al: The use and misuse of the fetal biophysical profile. *Am J Obstet Gynecol* 1987; 156:527.
6. Baskett TF: Gestational age and fetal biophysical assessment. *Am J Obstet Gynecol* 1988; 158:332.
7. Gross TL, Sokol RJ, Wilson MV, et al: Amniotic fluid phosphatidylglycerol: A potentially useful predictor of intrauterine growth retardation. *Am J Obstet Gynecol* 1981; 140:277.

14

Pediatric Management of Infants Small for Gestational Age

Avroy A. Fanaroff, M.B., F.R.C.P.E.
Maureen Hack, M.B., Ch.B.
Robert M. Kliegman, M.D.

The concept that there are different rates and patterns of intrauterine growth, first enunciated some 40 years ago, has facilitated recognition and anticipatory care of neonates with intrauterine growth retardation (IUGR). Recent sophistication and refinement of techniques for the evaluation of fetal growth, well-being, and maturity have resulted in the majority of such infants being recognized prior to delivery. This represents a quantum leap from a decade ago when less than one third of such infants were identified before labor and delivery, a time of great stress and danger for the growth-retarded fetus.[1]

Tables classifying infants according to birth weight and gestational age are utilized to determine whether growth has occurred at a normal, accelerated, or diminished rate in utero. At any gestational age the undergrown fetus demonstrates higher morbidity and mortality.[2] From a statistical point of view, infants born at any gestational age and weighing 2 SD below the mean are truly small for gestational age (SGA). However, because they share common clinical problems, all infants with birth weight at or below the 10th percentile for gestational age are regarded as SGA. Furthermore, many infants with birth weight above the 10th percentile will demonstrate evidence of weight loss and fall into the spectrum of the growth-retarded infant. Many synonyms including light for dates and intrauterine growth retardation are descriptive; however, common usage indicates preference for SGA.

Many conditions result in abnormal growth in utero. The cause and the timing, duration, and severity of the insult will modify the patterns of growth and hence the problems observed in the fetus and newborn infants. During the first trimester, global insults including perinatal infections (TORCH), ingested teratogens (such as anticonvulsants, alcohol, and anticoagulants), chromosomal abnormalities (trisomies 21, 18, and 13, and Turner's syndrome), and narcotic drug abuse initiate profound failure to growth of the fetus, resulting in a short infant of low birth weight, often with small head circumference and hence brain capacity. These infants with reduction in all growth parameters are referred to as having symmetric growth retardation.

Later onset of fetal growth failure results from disorders of the fetus or placenta or from maternal problems. Delivery of oxygen and nutrients is impeded by maternal or placental disorders in what is referred to as placental insufficiency. A dramatic effect of oxygen administration enhancing growth and correcting metabolic acidosis in a small group of growth-retarded infants was reported by Nicolaides et al.[3] These factors may become operative at variable times during pregnancy, resulting in less predictable effects on fetal growth. These disorders include, among others, maternal hypertension (preeclampsia and essential hypertension), smoking, malnutrition (undernutrition), and various forms of maternal vascular and renal diseases. They result in asymmetric growth retardation, which is characterized by weight at or below the 10th percentile, with length and head circumference above the 10th percentile. These infants have the potential for normal growth and development, yet are extremely vulnerable to perinatal asphyxia, which must be assiduously avoided. Perhaps equally vulnerable and often overlooked are the group of infants, frequently postterm, whose birth weight is above the 10th percentile but who have had recent weight loss in utero as evidenced by loose skinfolds as the result of loss of subcutaneous tissue.

Recent follow-up data suggest that IUGR as a consequence of malnutrition secondary to either maternal malnutrition or impaired uteroplacental transfer of nutrients is accompanied by a favorable outcome for the infant.[4] This prompted Warshaw[5] to question in a provocative editorial whether "IUGR resulting from restricted nutrient supply really represents pathology or is it a favorable adaptation of the fetus to maximize the prospects of good outcome? A strong case can be made for the latter." He further emphasizes that decreased fetal size with sparing of brain growth, acceleration of pulmonary maturation, and mild polycythemia, common features in the growth-retarded fetus, initially represent important adaptive strategies that become pathologic when deprivation becomes extreme and fetal distress supervenes. In the typical newborn with nutritionally induced IUGR, body proportions are asymmetric at birth, with brain growth and head circumference spared at the expense of both weight and linear growth. It is postulated that redistribution of the blood flow favors brain growth at the expense of the viscera and skeletal muscles (IUGR has been recognized in the fetus by studying the relationship between head and abdominal circumference ultrasonographically).

Another group of infants with disordered intrauterine growth includes those in whom specific genetic, inherited metabolic, or chromosome anomalies severely restrict growth potential. The products of multiple gestation and those with other specific syndromes and congenital malformations may also be SGA. In many infants no cause is identified for diminished growth; exposure to tobacco may be significant in this group. The variable causes and timing of the onset of the insults result in less predictability of growth, with both symmetric and asymmetric patterns observed. Nonetheless, more precise antenatal evaluation of fetal growth is permitting a more rational approach to the perinatal management of these complex problems and has resulted in a significant reduction in the incidence of stillbirth.

DELIVERY ROOM ASSESSMENT AND MANAGEMENT[6]

The timing of delivery of the growth-retarded infant remains controversial. It is important to gain an accurate picture of fetal growth, well-being, and maturity using a combination of biochemical, ultrasonographic, and biophysical tests. Fetal heart rate monitoring is indicated during labor, because there is a high incidence of fetal acidosis and distress. The neonatal resuscitation team should be present in the delivery room.

In pregnancies with compromised fetal growth, every effort must be made to avoid asphyxia and ensure an atraumatic delivery. The fetus is closely monitored during labor, and delivery is accomplished surgically if distress supervenes. When fetal compromise is established before labor, elective cesarean section is performed. Personnel skilled and experienced in neonatal resuscitation should be present at the delivery. A depressed infant with low Apgar scores should be anticipated. Resuscitative efforts designed to clear the airway, establish ventilation, support the circulation, and correct any metabolic acidosis are promptly initiated. The thermal environment should result in minimal oxygen consumption. If the amniotic fluid contains meconium, then the airway is cleared before delivery of the body, and subsequently the trachea is intubated and aspirated until clear.

Meconium aspiration syndrome is a frequent complication of fetal distress and has been associated with significant and unnecessarily high perinatal morbidity and mortality. The initial response to hypoxia is increased gastrointestinal motility, which together with relaxation of the anal sphincter releases meconium into the amniotic sac. This is most commonly observed beyond 35 weeks gestation. The presence of meconium in the amniotic fluid in association with abnormalities of fetal heart rate patterns and evidence of fetal acidosis as determined from the fetal scalp are clear evidence of fetal distress and indicate the forthcoming delivery of a depressed infant. Appropriate therapy to prevent meconium aspiration syndrome is complete clearance of the meconium from the oropharynx and tracheobronchial tree.

Vigorous stimulation and positive pressure ventilation may force meconium deep into the lungs and should only be performed after the airway has been thoroughly cleansed.

As the infant's head is delivered and prior to the first breath, the nasopharynx and oropharynx should be aspirated by the obstetrician using a DeLee catheter. Bulb suction is inadequate. After delivery the resuscitation proceeds with direct visualization and suctioning of the pharynx and trachea. Gregory et al.[7] noted that meconium was aspirated into the respiratory tract in 50% of all meconium-stained infants and that 10% of these infants have meconium below the vocal cords without evidence of meconium in the oropharynx. Based on this observation, it has been recommended that immediate endotracheal suctioning be done in all meconium-stained infants. Whereas these recommendations have been readily accepted for the infant born with thick meconium, controversy persists regarding the management of the lightly meconium-stained infant with good Apgar scores. A policy of universal intubation will result in unnecessary invasion of the upper airway in approximately 46% of infants. In skilled hands the complication rate is minimal, although vagal stimulation resulting in profound bradycardia will serve as a reminder that the procedure is not without risk. A change in technique of suctioning has been forced on health care providers because of the risk of acquired immune deficiency syndrome (AIDS). Whereas direct mouth-to-gauze suctioning of the endotracheal tube was commonplace, it is now essential that a remote technique of suctioning be used.

Studies are currently under way to determine whether it is necessary to intubate the trachea in infants with light meconium staining and high Apgar scores at 1 minute. Until these data are available, we will continue to recommend the combined obstetric-neonatal approach as outlined above for the prevention of meconium aspiration syndrome.

ASSESSMENT OF GESTATIONAL AGE

Once the initial transfer to extrauterine existence has been accomplished, the first order of business is to establish the birth weight/gestational age relationship.[8]

The clinical course and strategy for management are dependent on early identification of SGA infants. Thus it is essential to classify all infants as soon as possible as small, appropriate, or large for gestational age. Historically, gestational age is determined from a combination of the mother's dates and antenatal parameters including ultrasonographic examination when available, quickening, and detection of fetal heart. When the antenatal dating is not reliable, the neonatal assessment of gestational age is obtained from a combination of assessment of physical and neurologic characteristics according to the method of Dubowitz et al.[9] Ballard et al.[10] have produced an abbreviated version (see Table 1–1) that has become extremely popular and has been

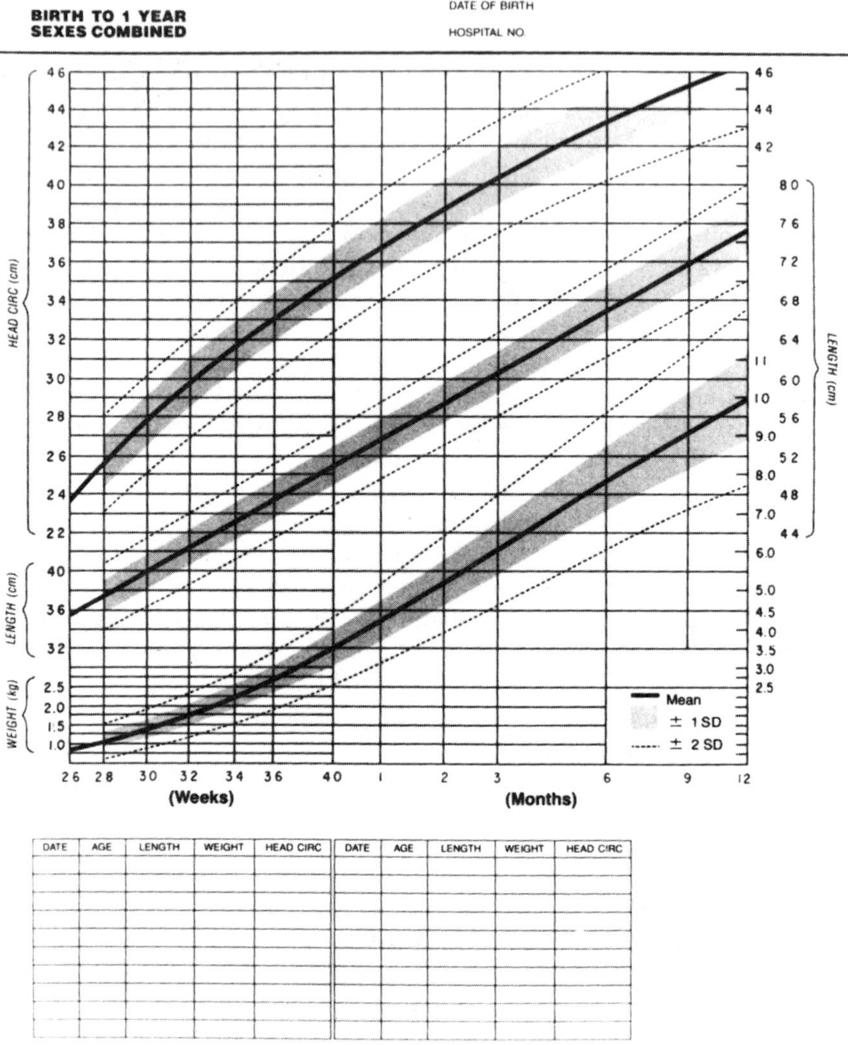

FIG 14–1.
Growth chart including weight, length, and head circumference. (Adapted from Babson SG, Benda GI: *J Pediatr* 1976; 89:814.)

statistically validated. It is important to plot the weight, length, and head circumference against normal standards and determine first if growth has been retarded, and if so, whether there is symmetric or asymmetric growth retardation. The Babson and Benda[11] charts (birth to 1 year) are extremely useful for this (Fig 14–1). If the infant is determined to be SGA, then the cause of the growth retardation must be sought and a management plan enacted to anticipate, prevent, and treat those conditions most prominent in these infants, as outlined in Table 14–1.

After the infant has been stabilized in the delivery room, a careful physical examination and additional measurements are necessary to confirm that the infant is SGA. For example, the ponderal index, which relates length to weight, is useful to further subclassify symmetric or asymmetric growth retardation and identify wasted infants. Physical and laboratory data are used to distinguish those infants with congenital malformations or congenital infections from those undergrown as a consequence of placental insufficiency. This is critical to determine the prognosis for the infant. The infant will then be closely monitored and any problems closely followed.

PHYSICAL EXAMINATION

SGA infants have relatively large heads for their wasted trunks and extremities, although approximately 50% of SGA infants with very low birth weight will have head circumferences below the 3rd percentile at birth. There is diminished subcutaneous tissue as evidenced by skinfold thickness determinations, and because of a lack of vernix, the skin is often desquamating and stained with meconium. Physical indicators of gestational age including sole creases, breast dimensions, and external appearance of the genitalia may be misleading because of variable effects of malnutrition, and the neurologic findings are usually more reliable and indicative of true gestational age. The neurologic examination may show accelerated maturation as a result of intrauterine stress and is not reliable in infants who have been severely asphyxiated.

Many postmature infants demonstrate evidence of late IUGR. Characteristically their length is at a higher percentile than their birth weight, and they have an anxious, alert appearance. The skin is dry, cracked, and wrinkled from loss of subcutaneous tissue, lacks vernix, and is often stained brownish green or yellow. The nails are long and the skull excessively firm. In common with SGA infants, perinatal complications include asphyxia, meconium aspiration syndrome, and hypoglycemia. In all infants a careful examination for malformations and evidence of congenital infections (see Table 14–1) is completed as soon as possible.

The clinical problems and the underlying physiologic mechanisms resulting in these problems in SGA infants are outlined in Table 14–2.[12] An understanding of the pathophysiology simplifies the clinical approach to these infants. It is worth noting that combinations of problems may occur in the same infant. Furthermore, the reserves of these SGA infants may have been taxed by the labor and delivery process, rendering them extremely vulnerable to physiologic deviations that would be readily compensated for by their appropriately grown counterparts. However, if all neonates are carefully examined and their birth weight/gestational age relationship diligently established, then the infants at risk are easily identified and the major problems

TABLE 14–1.
Comparison of Problems of SGA and Immature Newborn Infants*

	Immature AGA	Immature SGA	Mature SGA (Symmetric IUGR)	Mature SGA (Asymmetric IUGR)
Early weight change	5%-10% loss, then slow gain	5%-10% loss, then slow gain	5%-10% loss, then slow gain	≤5% loss, then rapid gain
Congenital infection	+	+ +	+ +	±
Respiratory problems	Hyaline membrane disease	Hyaline membrane disease	Unusual	Aspiration syndrome Pneumomediastinum Pneumothorax
Persistent fetal circulation	+	+	0	+ +
Apneic spells	+ + + +	+ + + +	0	0
Polycythemia	0	0	±	+ +
Hyperbilirubinemia	+ + + +	+ + + +	+	+ +
Hypoglycemia	+	+	+	+ + +
Hypocalcemia	+	+	±	+
Congenital malformation	±	+	+ +	±
Intracranial hemorrhage	+ + +	+ + +	±	+
Asphyxia	+ +	+ +	±	+ +
Growth (linear)	Normal	Subnormal (rare catch-up)	Subnormal (rare catch-up)	Normal
Neurobehavioral residua	+ + (mostly in very low birth weight infants)	+ + +	+ + +	+ (more if asphyxia is severe)

*Adapted from Sweet AY: Classification of the low-birth-weight infant, in Klaus MH, Fanaroff AA (eds): *Care of the High-Risk Neonate*, ed 3. Philadelphia, WB Saunders Co, 1986.

TABLE 14–2.
Perinatal Adaptive Problems*

Problem	Pathogenesis	Prevention
Perinatal asphyxia	↓ Placental reserve (insufficiency) ↓ Cardiac glycogen stores	Antepartum, intrapartum fetal heart rate monitoring
Meconium aspiration	Hypoxia/stress phenomenon	Oral-pharyngeal-tracheal suction
Fasting hypoglycemia	↓ Hepatic glycogen ↓ Gluconeogenesis	Early alimentation
Alimented hyperglycemia	"Starvation diabetes"	Avoid excessive carbohydrate loads
Polycythemia-hyperviscosity	Fetal hypoxia, ↑ erythropoietin Placental transfusion	Neonatal partial exchange transfusion
Temperature instability	↓ Adipose tissue ↑ Heat loss	Ensure neutral thermal environment
Pulmonary hemorrhage (rare)	Hypothermia, ↓ O_2/disseminated intravascular coagulation	Avoid cold stress, hypoxia
Immunodeficiency	"Malnutrition" effect	Unknown

*Adapted from Kliegman RM, Fanaroff AA: Developmental metabolism and nutrition, in Gregory GA (ed): *Pediatric Anesthesia*. New York, Churchill Livingstone, 1983.

anticipated and identified. Appropriate intervention can then be planned to ensure optimal outcome for the infant. The most common problems include asphyxia neonatorum, hypoglycemia, polycythemia/hyperviscosity, congenital malformations, and congenital infections. Jones and Roberton[13] at Cambridge reviewed the hospital course and outcome of 164 infants below the 5th percentile for gestation-specific birth weight and greater than or equal to 37 weeks' gestation. Finding a very low incidence of malformations (4%), congenital infections, or significant complications, they concluded that SGA infants of 37 or more weeks' gestation have few neonatal problems and do not require admission to the intensive care unit. They nonetheless still require close observation in the well-baby nursery. Nine (5%) infants did become hypoglycemic, but only one with associated respiratory distress required intravenous glucose.

HYPOGLYCEMIA

In the SGA infant the major problem initially of concern to the clinician is hypoglycemia. The clinical manifestations of hypoglycemia may be subtle, and because the neurologic consequences of sustained hypoglycemia are disastrous, it is imperative that all nursery personnel be alerted to this problem among SGA infants. A program whereby the blood glucose level is repeatedly screened if the infant is either small or large for gestational age can and must be effectively implemented. Hypoglycemia should be prevented or identified early enough to institute appropriate corrective measures.

SGA infants have diminished adipose tissue and low hepatic glycogen levels, rendering them vulnerable to fasting hypoglycemia. Although the growth-retarded infant initially has a lower metabolic rate than an appropriately grown peer, an attenuated gluconeogenesis response is observed. This can be corrected by intravenous or oral nutrient supplementation. Hypoglycemia is more common in male infants, discordant twins, and SGA infants, particularly in association with toxemia, asphyxia, polycythemia, and hypothermia.

The definition of hypoglycemia has traditionally been two whole blood glucose determinations below 30 mg/dl in the term infant during the first 72 hours of life and below 20 mg/dl on two occasions in the preterm infant. Most clinicians attempt to maintain the blood glucose level above 40 mg/dl. Normal values for blood glucose have been redefined by Srinivasan et al.[14] (Fig 14–2).

Inspection of these data indicates that the blood glucose level in the normal neonate does not drop below 40 mg/dl after 2 hours. We should strive to accomplish similar values in SGA and other infants at risk for hypoglycemia.

Hypoglycemia may have an insidious onset, which can be easily overlooked or present dramatically with the onset of seizures. A wide range of symptoms including apathy, poor feeding, apnea, high-pitched or weak cry, hypotonia, and eye rolling have all been attributed to hypoglycemia. These nonspecific symptoms may be present in normoglycemic neonates.

Hypoglycemia may have an early onset, within the first 1 to 2 hours after delivery, or appear later during the first week of life. Hypoglycemia should be anticipated in all SGA infants, and the blood glucose level monitored every 1 to 2 hours initially, and then every 2 to 4 hours until stabilized. Optimizing the environment to minimize energy needs, initiation of early feeding, and the liberal use of intravenous glucose infusions will prevent the majority of cases of hypoglycemia in SGA infants. Glucose is infused by pump at 4 to 9 mg/kg/min or greater if required. It is advisable to have a second intravenous line in place to obviate discontinuation of the infusion if the line becomes infiltrated.

If the infant has symptoms of hypoglycemia, a minibolus of 2 ml/kg 10% aqueous dextrose solution should be infused rapidly and followed by an infusion at 8 mg/kg/min, monitoring the blood glucose level every 30 minutes. The rate may be increased in 2 mg/kg/min increments to achieve normoglycemia.

Symptomatic neonatal hypoglycemia is a serious disorder requiring prompt recognition and intervention to prevent permanent CNS sequelae. Thirty to 50% of symptomatic hypoglycemic neonates may subsequently demonstrate neurologic impairment.

Treatment of Hypoglycemia[15]

The following regimen is used to treat hypoglycemia:

1. Minibolus 2 ml/kg 10% aqueous dextrose solution over 1 minute.
2. Follow with 8 mg/kg/min 10% dextrose (4.8 ml/kg/hr, 115 ml/kg/24 hr).
3. Maintain two intravenous lines.
4. Start oral feeds early.
5. If glucose level is still low, increase stepwise to 12 to 14 mg/kg/min 10% dextrose.
6. Start steroids if hypoglycemia persists or recurs.
7. Closely monitor glucose concentration.

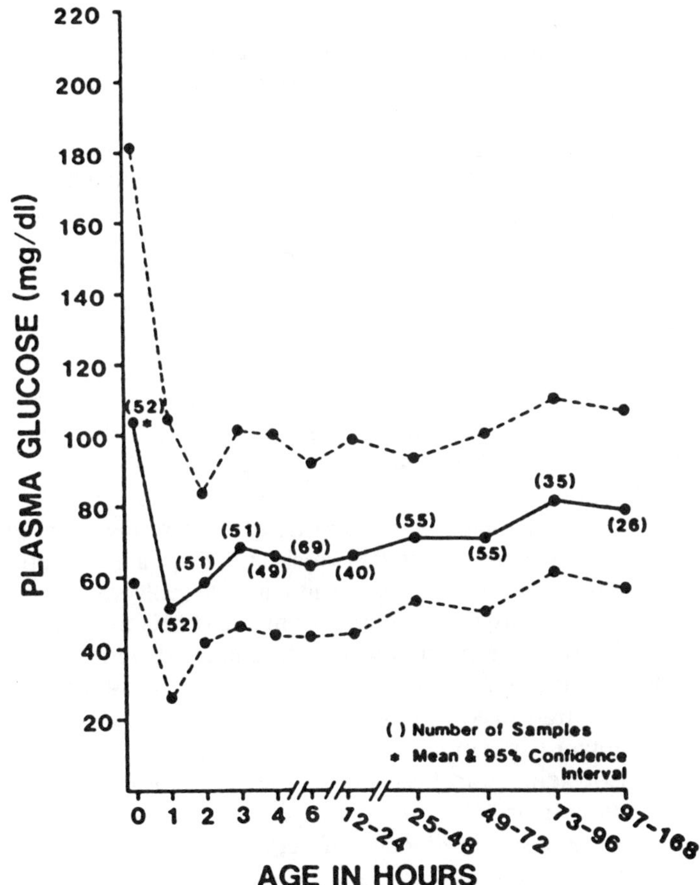

FIG 14–2.
Predicted plasma glucose values during first week of life in healthy term neonates appropriate for gestational age. (From Srinivasan G, et al: *J Pediatr* 1986; 109:114. Used by permission.)

RESPIRATORY DIFFICULTIES

Term and post-term SGA infants are prone to intrauterine asphyxia and passage of meconium in utero. Meconium may be aspirated into the lungs because asphyxiated infants will commence gasping in utero. The combined perinatal approach including oropharyngeal suction by the obstetrician as soon as the head has been delivered and endotracheal intubation and suctioning by the pediatrician after delivery has significantly reduced both the morbidity and mortality from meconium aspiration syndrome. There remain, however, a few infants who have presumably had prolonged hypoxemia in utero. These infants have a combination of meconium aspiration and persistence of the fetal circulation. Their pulmonary vasculature is abnormal, with muscular layers persisting in the pulmonary arterioles all the way to the alveoli. This results in significant pulmonary hypertension that presents an extremely difficult clinical problem.

Current goals of management are minimal handling of the infants, liberal use of oxygen, alkalinization of the blood predominantly with hyperventilation and bicarbonate therapy, and the occasional use of agents such as tolazoline to reduce pulmonary hypertension. Extracorporeal membrane oxygenation has been used in infants in whom a mortality rate of 80% or greater has been predicted from persistence of poor blood gases. Preliminary results are encouraging.

POLYCYTHEMIA

Polycythemia is defined by venous hematocrit above 65%. In appropriately grown newborns the incidence is approximately 4%, rising to 18% to 45% in SGA infants. The high hematocrit is thought to be the result of intrauterine hypoxia stimulating erythropoietin, but may also be secondary to twin-to-twin transfusion. Infants with high hematocrit values may have hyperviscosity and reduced red cell deformability. They are susceptible to thrombotic complications. Symptoms attributable to polycythemia include respiratory distress, lethargy, jitteriness, edema, and priapism. Infants with polycythemia are also more prone to hypoglycemia and jaundice.

The tendency has been to empirically reduce the hematocrit by means of partial exchange transfusion if the value is greater than 70%, or greater than 65% if the infant has symptoms.

The partial isovolemic transfusion most effectively lowers the viscosity if normal saline solution or 5% albumin is used. The exchange volume necessary to achieve the desired reduction of hematocrit to approximately 55% is calculated as follows:

$$\frac{\text{Volume (ml)} = \text{Blood volume x (Hct1} - \text{Hct2)}}{\text{Hct1}}$$

where Hct1 = initial hematocrit and Hct2 = desired hematocrit.

Current indications for intervention in neonates with polycythemia remain largely empirical extrapolations from studies of blood viscosity. Some recent studies indicate that the whole blood viscosity is lower in neonates than in adults at every level of hematocrit and that this is the result of a lower plasma viscosity. It is important to take into account hematocrit and total plasma proteins in deriving microviscosity. Intervention is not undertaken lightly. The major risk of the partial exchange transfusion is the increased incidence of bowel necrosis and necrotizing enterocolitis.

In a recent study Murphy et al.[16] evaluated the cardiac function in infants with polycythemia. M-mode echocardiograms were performed before and after a partial exchange transfusion and repeated 48 hours later. The polycythemic infants with presumed blood hyperviscosity had slower heart rates and findings consistent with elevated pulmonary vascular resistance. The elevated right ventricular pre-ejection/right ventricular ejection time corrected with the partial exchange. An unexplained fractional shortening was noted in the polycythemic infants 48 hours after the exchange.

FOLLOW-UP[1, 4, 17-19]

Follow-up programs have traditionally been considered the less glamorous aspect of perinatal centers. Nonetheless, follow-up remains a cornerstone of the perinatal puzzle, the yardstick whereby perinatal care may be evaluated and the true measure of any new therapeutic intervention. It is particularly important to observe all infants with evidence of IUGR or asphyxia, because they represent a group at particularly high risk for poor neurodevelopmental outcome.

The long-term prognosis for SGA infants has slowly emerged. In view of the many variables affecting growth and development and the heterogenous group of infants defined as SGA, it is not surprising that reports of outcome range from extremely optimistic to depressingly pessimistic. The ultimate outcome is dependent on the cause of the aberrant growth, including the presence of congenital infections or malformations, the timing and duration of the insult, severity of growth retardation, degree of intrauterine or postnatal asphyxia, postnatal course, and above all the socioeconomic status of the family. Recent reports identify and attempt to control these variables, facilitating interpretation of the results.

Very few preterm infants who are SGA at birth catch up in growth during the neonatal period as superimposed on their intrauterine causes of growth failure; they have a variety of neonatal problems that further affect growth. In our experience, 91% of SGA infants will still be <2 SD below the norm at 40 weeks corrected age. Varying patterns of growth are observed during the first year of life, with the most rapid catch-up growth occurring during this period. Some infants who failed to grow during the neonatal period will demonstrate an accelerated growth velocity and catch up; others may demonstrate a normal growth velocity but remain small and never catch up; few have a low growth velocity and frankly fail to thrive. Growth during infancy is influenced by many factors, including the persistence of perinatal problems such as bronchopulmonary dysplasia, necrotizing enterocolitis, cholestasis, and malabsorption. Additional factors influencing growth include the need for rehospitalization, caretaking disorders, and feeding problems in children with neurologic impairment. SGA infants rarely catch up in weight after the first year, and in our experience at 3 years some 50% of SGA infants still have subnormal weight (Fig 14–3). There is very little evidence in the literature to support the concept that these infants will catch up later in life. Caretakers must thus make every effort during the first year of life to ensure maximal nutritional support and to utilize nutritional and nonnutritive techniques to optimize caloric utilization.

It is important to follow the growth of the head, because this is indicative of brain size and correlates well with intellectual development. It is noteworthy that the SGA infant with a small head at birth may still have normal development. Some 50% of SGA infants will have a small head circumference at birth; catch-up indicates a good outlook. At times it is difficult to distinguish catch-up head growth from hydrocephalus, and we are using ultrasonography liberally to detect, among other things, congenital or acquired anatomic abnormalities, evidence of bleeding, and ventricular size. Computed tomography is used to clarify suspect lesions.

The timing, duration, and cause of the IUGR together with the degree of catch-up growth determine the outcome of both term and preterm growth-retarded infants. The outcome reports of SGA term infants have varied. Normal IQ predominates; however, language delay, behavioral problems, and potential school difficulties despite normal IQ are emerging as significant problems. As indicated, early reports on SGA preterm infants were devastating and depressing. Recent reports excluding infants with congenital infections and major malformations have not found significant differences between SGA and appropriately grown preterm infants. This has been attributed to many factors, including earlier recognition, more precise intrauterine monitoring, appropriate delivery with avoidance of asphyxia and trauma, avoidance of hypoglycemia, and improved postnatal nutrition. SGA infants, nonetheless, do appear to exhibit more minor neurologic abnormalities. Infants at greatest risk for poor neurodevelopmental outcome include those weighing 1 kg or less at birth, those with asphyxia and seizures in the neonatal period, those with congenital infections and major malformations, and those who do not catch up in any of the growth parameters.

The follow-up of the SGA infant presents a continuing challenge. All infants should be considered at risk, and every effort should be made by caretakers to ensure that these infants are presented with all the available resources at the medical center so that they can achieve their maximum potential.

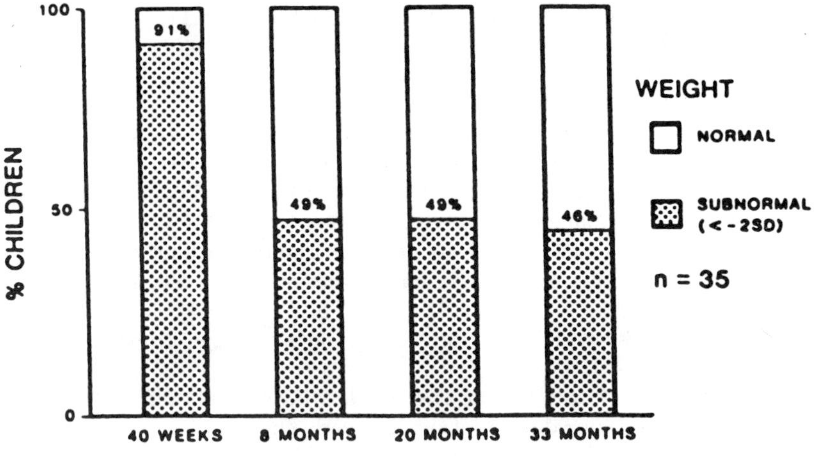

FIG 14–3.
Infant weight in the population of SGA neonates. (From Hack M, Fanaroff AA: *Clin Obstet Gynecol* 1984; 27:647. Used by permission.)

REFERENCES

1. Drillien C: The small for dates infants: Etiology and prognosis. *Pediatr Clin North Am* 1970; 17:9.
2. Koops BL, Møorgan LJ, Battaglia FC: Neonatal mortality risk in relation to birth weight and gestational age: Update. *J Pediatr* 1982; 101:969.
3. Nicolaides KH, Bradley RJ, Soothill PW, et al: Maternal oxygen therapy for intrauterine growth retardation. *Lancet* 1987; 1:942.
4. Hack M, Fanaroff AA: The outcome of growth failure associated with preterm birth. *Clin Obstet Gynecol* 1984; 27:647.
5. Warshaw JB: Intrauterine growth retardation: Adaptation or pathology? Commentary. *Pediatrics* 1985; 76:998.
6. Martin RJ, Fanaroff AA: Delivery room management of the very low birthweight infant. *Clin Obstet Gynecol* 1984; 27:636.
7. Gregory G, Gooding C, Phibbs R, et al: Meconium aspiration in infants — A prospective study. *J Pediatr* 1974; 85:848.
8. Sweet AY: Classification of the low-birth-weight infant, in Klaus MH, Fanaroff AA (eds): *Care of the High-Risk Neonate*, ed 3. Philadelphia, WB Saunders Co, 1986.
9. Dubowitz L, Dubowitz V, Goldberg C: Clinical assessment of gestational age in the newborn infant. *J Pediatr* 1970; 77:1.
10. Ballard JL, Novak KK, Driver M: A simplified score for assessment of fetal maturation of newly born infants. *J Pediatr* 1979; 95:769.
11. Babson SG, Benda GI: Growth graphs for the clinical assessment of infants of varying gestational age. *J Pediatr* 1976; 89:814.

12. Kliegman RM, Fanaroff AA: Developmental metabolism and nutrition, in Gregory GA (ed): *Pediatric Anesthesia*. New York, Churchill Livingstone, 1983.
13. Jones RAK, Roberton NRC: Small for dates babies: Are they really a problem? *Arch Dis Child* 1986; 61:877.
14. Srinivasan G, Pildes RS, Cattamanchi G, et al: Plasma glucose values in normal neonates: A new look. *J Pediatr* 1986; 109:114.
15. Pildes RS, Lilien LD: Carbohydrate disorders, in Fanaroff AA, Martin RJ (eds): *Neonatal-Perinatal Medicine*. St. Louis, CV Mosby Co, 1987.
16. Murphy DJ Jr, Reller MD, Meyer RA, et al: Left ventricular function in normal newborn infants and asymptomatic infants with neonatal polycythemia. *Am Heart J* 1986; 112:542.
17. Fitzhardinge P, Steven E: The small for dates infant. I: Later growth patterns. *Pediatrics* 1972; 49:671.
18. Hack M, Caron B, Rivers A, et al: The very low birth weight infant: The broader spectrum of morbidity during infancy and early childhood. *J Dev Behav Pediatr* 1983; 4:243.
19. Walther FJ, Ramaekers LHJ: Neonatal morbidity of SGA infants in relation to their nutritional status at birth. *Acta Paediatr Scand* 1982; 71:437.

15

Frontiers in Fetal Therapy

Mark I. Evans, M.D.
Robert J. Sokol, M.D.

Other chapters in this volume detail many of the practical aspects of the diagnosis and antepartum and intrapartum management of intrauterine growth retardation (IUGR) in current appropriate clinical practice.

In this chapter we will attempt to distance ourselves to some extent from what is currently known about intrauterine growth retardation (IUGR) and take a critical look at our limited concepts of etiology and pathogenesis underlying diagnostic and therapeutic methods. We will try to think beyond the currently recommended methods for diagnosis and therapy of IUGR to a time when we will have a much better idea of what we are really attempting to diagnose and treat, leading to the possibility for innovative intrauterine treatment of IUGR. Indeed, this brief chapter could most appropriately be entitled "Speculations about IUGR."

PROBLEMS WITH CURRENT DIAGNOSIS AND THERAPY

The problems with definition of IUGR as an overall concept and with regard to deciding which specific fetuses should be termed growth retarded contribute significantly to the diagnostic dilemma often presented by the antenatal detection of the growth-retarded fetus.[1,2] Currently and most typically, birth weight at less than the 10th percentile or at less than the tenth percentile for gestational age is used as a marker for IUGR. The terms "small for gestational age" and "intrauterine growth retarded" are often used nearly interchangeably, obfuscating the fact that these two concepts are distinct; confusing the two leads to both false positive and false negative results.

A 28-year-old, white, 6 ft, 150 lb gravida 2 para 1 from an upper socioeconomic group without any significant prenatal risk factors might be expected to be delivered of an infant of considerably greater weight at full term than the usual average of around 3,250 gm. The *expected* weight of such an infant might be closer to 3,800 gm, for example. Thus if the infant weighs, say 2,900 gm, certainly greater than the 10th percentile at 40 weeks gestation and thus not small for gestational age by definition, that infant may still be severely growth retarded. Currently there is no practical technology available to effectively deal with such a situation, on either a research or a clinical basis. A 2,500 gm infant born at full term to a 4 ft 10 inch primigravida without antenatal risks highlights the situation in which the infant is, by definition, small for gestational age but may not be growth retarded in the pathologic sense. Until we are able to reliably calculate expected fetal size or, even better, growth rates based on individual patient characteristics and to obtain reliable estimates of observed fetal growth and size, our ability to choose cases for appropriate medical intervention will remain distinctly limited.

From the perspective of treatment of IUGR, another critical limiting factor is a fundamental dearth of insightful hypotheses as to its most common causes and pathophysiologic mechanisms. Because of this limitation, typical treatment plans at this time are empiric rather than scientifically based and are almost, by definition, closer to a shotgun approach, rather than a magic bullet. Thus, therapy to this time has been principally based on treating symptoms rather than causes. Prenatal treatment of IUGR is similar to that of diabetes mellitus in the 1960s. Prior to our understanding of the importance of euglycemia, management was based on the concept of balancing the risks of continued intrauterine existence with the attendant risk of unpredictable fetal death, and preterm delivery with the risk of prematurity related neonatal death. The key at that time was the timing of delivery, perhaps the most nonspecific of all obstetric interventions, though patient management was directed by the most advanced concepts available given the very limited understanding of the disorder. Various therapeutic interventions for IUGR are currently carried out similarly independent of knowledge of the cause of IUGR. What emerges is an appreciation of our need for new pathophysiologic and etiologic concepts. "Are there any?"

CONCEPTS

As new ways of thinking about the cause and pathogenesis of IUGR and resulting new classifications are delineated, it will be possible to relate potential fetal therapies to the specific problem at hand, leading to a gradual shift from empiric to rational therapy. Current work must focus on elucidating such differences. It is reasonable to hypothesize that just as different known diseases are often associated with different steps of the biochemical pathway, there are also specifically different types of IUGR, related to maternal nutrient uptake, delivery to the placenta, placental transport and exchange, fetal blood flow, and fetal nutrient metabolism. These cannot be differentiated currently. In our opinion the currently used distinction between symmetric and asymmetric growth retardation is not useful for this purpose and may actually cloud the situation further. IUGR should be seen as a "final common pathway"[3] rather than a specific disease. It is a detectable sign of maternofetal pathophysiology.

An alternative concept is based on the classic concept of the homeostasis of the internal milieu. From this perspective IUGR is a homeostatic mechanism teleologically aimed at preserving the fetus (except in genetic diseases) in which there is limited potential. As such, IUGR would not be considered a disease but an adaptation to limitation of supply in the broadest sense.

A competing concept of IUGR would postulate some inherent fetal placental defect that does not induce normal circulatory and metabolic change in the mother, in turn reducing oxygen and nutrient delivery to the fetus. It is easy to see how such a concept would lead to a different approach to therapy than that presented above. Indeed, either or both concepts may be applicable to an individual fetus, so that an additional problem becomes differentiating appropriate conceptual models for this perinatal problem.

In the remainder of this chapter we make certain assumptions about technologic advances that may make it possible in the near future to subdivide nongenetic IUGR into several major etiologic components:

1. Deficient maternal substrate because of maternal starvation.
2. Inadequate maternal vasculature with decreased uterine blood flow.
3. Abnormal maternofetal placental exchange with diminished transfer of otherwise adequately available nutrients.

The field of "fetal therapy" is in its own infancy.[4] Although heroic surgical interventions have been given notoriety in both the scientific and lay presses, it is likely that less glamorous, more effective pharmacologic procedures will become the mainstay of fetal therapy over the next two decades. Most fetal therapeutic attempts to date have been aimed at altering the course of either genetic disorders or nonspecific congenital malformations. In the following sections we explore some possibilities of positively influencing fetal growth rather than correcting the negative consequences of congenital anomalies.

POTENTIAL TREATMENT APPROACHES

For those types of IUGR secondary to an extrinsic deficiency of nutrient delivery to the fetus, it may be possible in a limited number of situations to bypass inefficient delivery systems and replace specific deficient elements or alter metabolic functions. Realistically, however, for intrinsic fetal defects, such as trisomy 18, there is no hope in the foreseeable future of being able to correct the massive multisystem derangements. Perhaps our grandchildren will have the capability to address such issues or the wisdom to know whether it would be worth the effort.

Deficient Maternal Substrates

There have been numerous attempts to supplement maternal deficiencies.[5–8] Most attempts have been in patients with specific maternal conditions such as severe maternal gastrointestinal disorders, in which complete gastrointestinal rest is necessary. Hyperalimentation has been used in such patients, with both recovery of normal gastrointestinal function for the mother and apparently adequate nutrition for the fetus. Though data are still relatively limited, interesting possibilities are raised for the treatment of the mother who does not necessarily have significant nutritional or metabolic deprivation. Even for the mother who is medically well but whose fetus is growth retarded, hyperalimentation could conceivably remediate inadequate fetal nutrition. We are aware of one unpublished attempt to place an indwelling catheter to deliver amino acids to the fetus. However, we are unaware of any rigorous efforts to provide hyperalimentation to the fetus in the presence of apparently adequate maternal nutrition. What is needed is a clinical trial of defined nutrients given intravenously to the mother and another trial of direct injections to the fetus. Such studies might well help define the exact nature of deficiency as being maternal, placental, or fetal and also test an essentially pharmacologic treatment for fetal malnutrition. Direct injections, now technically possible by percutaneous umbilical cord access, would have the further advantage of bypassing the metabolic utilization of nutrients by both the mother and the placenta.

As noted, in probably the majority of fetuses IUGR is a function of restricted access to nutrients rather than an intrinsic defect of potential.[9] Thus at a simplistic level it may be theoretically possible to compensate for some of the deficiencies. It is worth stressing again, however, that under circumstances of diminished availability of nutrients or capability to process them, it is teleologically advantageous for the fetus to be small. As obstetricians we tend to focus our attention on the vulnerability of the IUGR fetus at term. What we often fail to appreciate is that slow growth may be the only reason that the fetus has survived at all.

Intraamniotic and intrafetal injections of various substances have been attempted. For example, IUGR has been "treated" with long-term amino acid infusion.[10] This suggests the possibility of intraamniotic nutrient injection. Although amniocentesis in the third trimester is very safe in experienced hands, it seems unlikely, except in the most dire circumstances, that repeated procedures that would probably be necessary to support intrauterine nutrition would be clinically practicable. Furthermore, there is then a question of fetal uptake by swallowing of amniotic fluid. A potential alternative to ensure appropriate uptake would be fetal umbilical catheterization. At present the procedure is relatively risky, with a 1% to 3% fetal mortality rate in the most experienced hands. Nonetheless, in the future repeated access to umbilical vessels or long-term catheterization of a vessel may make this a more efficient mechanism of ensuring fetal systemic absorption in certain situations.

Plasma Volume Expansion

It has been appreciated for about a decade that one of the hallmarks of IUGR is inadequate plasma volume expansion.[11,12] Furthermore, studies have suggested that the rate of plasma volume expansion is proportional to the initial prepregnancy maternal plasma volume.[12] Prepregnancy volumes are correlated with initial osmotic and oncotic pressure, and in maternal malnutrition we would expect the osmotic and oncotic forces of the mother to be below normal, thus correlating with the poor expansion of pregnancy.[13] There is no consensus, however, as to whether poor plasma volume expansion is a cause or an effect of IUGR.

To date, attempts at maternal plasma volume expansion have been limited, because albumin is expensive and because concerns of potential transfer of infectious diseases, such as acquired immune deficiency syndrome (AIDS), have no doubt dampened the enthusiasm of potential investigators. Artificial plasma components continue under development and might have a role as plasma volume expanders in pregnancy. It may be possible to artificially and, it is hoped, more than transiently increase maternal plasma volume either before or in very early pregnancy. If so, it might be possible to prevent the initiation of the IUGR sequence in selected patients. It must be stressed that this is highly speculative.

Diminished Placental Transfer

Inefficient maternofetal nutrient passage can be seen in several situations. For example, in abruptio placenta the conduit for passage between the maternal and fetal sides can be disrupted. Placenta previa is a determinant of IUGR because both the site and the efficiency of attachment are less than optimal.[14] Furthermore, fetoplacental surface interactions can be further reduced by the loss of the cervical area and the greater tendency for prenatal bleeding to separate maternal from fetal circulations. Such data have been collected in animal models, although quantitative human data are limited. Perhaps with advances in ultrasonography it may be possible to collect such data in the future.

The issue of aberrant placental transfer raises perhaps the most esoteric and futuristic possibilities to be considered here. Ultimately an artificial placenta will be invented, but this may be 10, 20, or 100 years off. Just as the iron lung made possible the continued existence of patients with pulmonary and neuromuscular disorders in the 1940s and 1950s, for the fetus of the 1990s with inadequate oxygenation it may be possible to temporize delivery by using a more efficient artificial system when the biologic placenta can no longer do the job, along the lines of "intrauterine extracorporeal membrane oxygenation." Using an extracorporeal membrane oxygenator with dialysis-type equipment, it may be possible to provide for the premature growth-retarded fetus adequate oxygenation, sustenance, and clearance of metabolic wastes to allow it to develop its own capabilities when the maternal system has failed. Further, the advent of recombinant DNA technology may eventually permit in utero bone marrow transplantation of genes to promote fetal metabolism of limited nutrients. Possibilities might include transplantation of growth-promoting genes.[15] As more specific causes of IUGR become clear and control of fetal growth better understood, recombinant genes to promote certain enzymatic reactions will become possible.

CONCLUSIONS

New frontiers in fetal therapy of IUGR are embryonic. Without the better delineation of pathogeneses, treatments can only be empiric and symptomatic. However, as knowledge of IUGR becomes more specific, tailor-made solutions to specific problems should be more reasonably expected. It is entirely possible that for the vast majority of growth-retarded fetuses specific therapy may be decades off. However, one by one we can expect many of the more esoteric and specifically delineated causes of IUGR to become amenable to possible treatment.

It is likely that as we define the causes of IUGR, therapies will be tailored to the individual mechanism. It is not likely that genetic or infectious causes will be readily treatable. Yet we believe that the crux of future developments will be increasing sophistication of diagnosis, including the use of new molecular genetic techniques. Improved biologic models and diagnostic methods will finally allow therapies to move from an empiric to a rational basis.

REFERENCES

1. Seeds JW: Impaired fetal growth: Definition and clinical diagnosis. *Obstet Gynecol* 1984; 64:303.
2. Wilcox AJ: Intrauterine growth retardation: Beyond birth weight criteria. *Early Hum Dev* 1983; 8:189.
3. Evans MI, Lin CC: Normal fetal growth, in Lin CC, Evans MI (eds): *Intrauterine Growth Retardation.* New York, McGraw-Hill Book Co, 1984, pp 17–43.
4. Schulman JD (ed): Fetal Therapy. *Clin Obstet Gynecol* 1986; 29:481–614.
5. Hew LR, Deitel M: Total parenteral nutrition in gynecology and obstetrics. *Obstet Gynecol* 1980; 55:464.

6. Cox KL, Byrne WJ, Ament ME: Home total parenteral nutrition during pregnancy: A case report. *J Parent Enter Nutr* 1981; 5:246.
7. Weinberg RB, Sitrin MD, Adkins G, et al: The treatment of hyperlipidemic pancreatitis in pregnancy with total parenteral nutrition. *Gastroenterology* 1982; 83:1300.
8. Webb GA: The use of hyperalimentation and chemotherapy in pregnancy: A case report. *Am J Obstet Gynecol* 1980; 137:263.
9. Lin CC, Evans MI: Introduction, in Lin CC, Evans MI (eds): *Intrauterine Growth Retardation.* New York, McGraw-Hill Book Co, 1984, pp 1–13.
10. Saling J: Treatment of IUGR with amino acid infusion. Presented at Kings College Symposium on Prenatal Diagnosis and Fetal Therapy, London, November 1986.
11. Croall J, Sheriff S, Matthews J: Nonpregnancy maternal plasma volume expansion in pregnant rats. *J Nutr* 1979; 11:1887.
12. Hytten FE, Leitch I: *The Physiology of Human Pregnancy,* ed 2. Oxford, Blackwell Scientific Publications, 1971.
13. Evans MI, Lin CC: Retarded fetal growth, in Lin CC, Evans MI (eds): *Intrauterine Growth Retardation.* New York, McGraw-Hill Book Co, 1984, pp 65–67.
14. Evans MI, Lin CC: Retarded fetal growth, in Lin CC, Evans MI (eds): *Intrauterine Growth Retardation.* New York, McGraw-Hill Book Co, 1984, pp 60–61.
15. Palmiter RD, Brinster RL, Hammer RE, et al: Dramatic growth of mice that develop from eggs microjected with metallothionein–growth hormone fusion genes. *Nature* 1982; 300:611.

16

Problems in Practical Diagnosis and Management of Intrauterine Growth Retardation: Perinatal Rounds

Robert J. Sokol, M.D.
Richard A. Bronsteen, M.D.
Mitchell P. Dombrowski, M.D.
Federico G. Mariona, M.D.

This chapter has an entirely different format from those preceding it in this book. In this chapter we apply some of the information presented in previous chapters to the discussion of real patient care problems. The format we have chosen mimics in print what might occur on "perinatal" or "high-risk" rounds, with four perinatologists in attendance. Each of these perinatologists is experienced in the diagnosis and management of pregnancies complicated by intrauterine growth retardation (IUGR). Each has contributed in writing independently of the others, so you will no doubt note some repetition and disagreement. In some areas you may disagree as well — as in real rounds!

PATIENT 1

> A 24-year-old, gravida 3 para 2 oriental woman came to her initial prenatal visit with unknown menstrual dates. She denied any problems with the pregnancy other than occasional nausea and vomiting. Previous medical history was normal except for several episodes of cystitis. The patient smoked one pack of cigarettes per day and consumed alcohol sparingly. She had previously given birth to two singleton term infants weighing 2,381 and 2,523 gm, respectively. Both were delivered by uncomplicated vaginal delivery and are currently well. Her prepregnancy weight was 98 lb.

DR. SOKOL: A few points about this patient's history are worth comment. That she has unknown menstrual dates isn't the least unusual at our institution. This is always a problem, but particularly with regard to the diagnosis of IUGR. The patient has two obvious historical risks for IUGR. She is a smoker and she weighs less than 100 lb; these two factors alone, in conjunction with her unknown menstrual history, are clear indications for obtaining a sonographic scan as soon as possible to "nail down" gestational duration as reliably as possible.

Something else that is absolutely crucial in this history is that this woman has had two small infants. Because the implications for the current pregnancy are different if these were preterm infants or if they were small for gestational age (SGA), it is crucial for the clinician to attempt to make this determination historically. Here is a trick that I have found useful in the office: Patients seldom think in terms of weeks of gestation. They may know they delivered in the eighth month or the ninth month, but they seldom know whether they delivered at 36 weeks or 39 weeks. I have been impressed, however, that most multiparas remember their due dates from previous pregnancies, and of course they know the birth dates of their children. In that way it is possible for the clinician to calculate the weeks of gestation at birth. Alternatively, a woman may not remember the exact dates, but she will almost surely remember that she delivered 4 weeks early or 2 weeks late, for example. From weeks of gestation and birth weight, and using an appropriate birth weight percentile chart (in this case a chart standardized for sea level), the clinician can calculate birth weight percentiles. Birth weight of this patient's first child was at approximately the 2nd percentile, and of her second child at approximately the 4th birth weight percentile. Previous SGA birth is one of the most predictive factors of another SGA birth, with a single previous SGA birth increasing the risk for SGA birth in the current pregnancy something in the range of two- to threefold.

Two final observations: With two previous SGA births, low maternal weight, and current smoking, this patient is at very high risk for the birth of an SGA infant in the current pregnancy. She is going to require very close antepartum supervision. Second, I have the clinical suspicion that previous birth weight percentiles as low as in this patient's previous children, assuming 40-week gestations, are more consistent with some type of asymmetric growth problem, such as malnutrition or vascular disease, than with these infants being only constitutionally small.

The pertinent physical findings at first visit included weight 103 lb, height 152 cm, and blood pressure 100/60 mm Hg. Findings of cardiac and pulmonary examinations were normal. The uterine fundal height was 20 cm, and fetal heart tones were auscultated with a fetoscope. Routine laboratory findings included a negative antibody screen, blood type B+, negative rubella titer, hematocrit 34%, and a normal Papanicolaou smear. Urine and gonococcal cultures were negative, and the VDRL nonreactive. An ultrasound examination performed at this time revealed a 20-week singleton fetus by biparietal diameter, femur length, and abdominal circumference. Amniotic fluid volume was normal. The placenta was fundal and grade 0.

The patient's weight gain and blood pressures through the second and early third trimesters were appropriate. Uterine fundal height measurements were consistent with dates (by initial ultrasound study) until 30 weeks gestation. However, from 30 to 34 weeks gestation the fundal height increased by only 1 cm. Therefore IUGR was suspected clinically on the basis of poor or no uterine growth over 4 weeks and size less than expected for dates. A repeat ultrasound revealed a fetus that was 32 weeks by biparietal diameter and femur length and 31 weeks by abdominal circumference.

DR. MARIONA: In spite of the positive findings of Belizán et al.,[1] who utilized fundal height measurements for the clinical diagnosis of IUGR, more recent studies have failed to document this technique as a reliable screening tool for IUGR. In this case fundal height measurements are further limited by the lack of a specific reference for the patient's ethnic group and body habitus.

DR. BRONSTEEN: Although this repeated study is within the expected third-trimester sonographic range of ±3 weeks, the interval growth in the 14 weeks from the initial study is suboptimal. Also, the increased head/abdomen circumference ratio is suggestive of asymmetric growth retardation, although the criteria of more than 2 SD above the mean has not been attained. At this point both clinical and sonographic evidence is suggestive but not diagnostic for IUGR.

DR. SOKOL: Dr. Bronsteen hints at an important point. We usually consider that a minimum interval of 3 weeks between ultrasound examinations in the third trimester is necessary to accurately assess fetal growth. If the patient, however, has had more than one previous ultrasound study, we can calculate interval growth from the previous to the current study rather than from the last to the current ultrasound study. Clinical experience indicates that this is often a useful approach providing increased sensitivity in diagnosis.

On the day after the second ultrasound examination amniocentesis was performed and 10 ml clear amniotic fluid was aspirated. Analysis of the fluid revealed a mature L/S ratio and trace amounts of phosphatidylglycerol.

DR. BRONSTEEN: Gross et al.[2,3] have shown that acceleration of fetal lung maturity may be predictive of growth retardation.

DR. DOMBROWSKI: Although amniocentesis may be helpful in the diagnosis and management of IUGR, in this case an argument against the procedure could be made. An invasive procedure such as amniocentesis should not be performed unless the potential benefits outweigh the potential complications and the clinician is prepared to act on the information gained by the procedure. Hypothetically, if the physician is willing to deliver a fetus with suspected IUGR on the basis of mature or meconium-stained amniotic fluid, then amniocentesis may be indicated. However, if there is adequate fluid volume, continued interval growth, and reassuring antenatal testing, then delivery before 37 weeks is probably not indicated, even with mature fluid. In a study by Perry et al.,[4] growth-retarded infants had a better outcome when delivered between 38 and 42 weeks, compared with those delivered between 28 and 37 weeks.

DR. BRONSTEEN: As noted, mature amniotic fluid fetal lung indices at or before 34 weeks gestation raise suspicions of IUGR. Do mature lung indices and growth retardation mandate immediate delivery? Or is it better for the fetus to remain in the compromised uterine environment in an effort to avoid the added complications of prematurity to those of growth retardation? Growth-retarded fetuses have been shown to experience developmental and neurologic problems on follow-up.[5,6] Optimal delivery time involves balancing the risks of prematurity with those of continued stay in a compromised intrauterine environment.

Several studies have shown antenatal fetal heart rate testing to be predictive of fetal morbidity and mortality.[7,8] As with the results of antenatal testing for other high-risk patients, reassuring antenatal testing in growth retardation correlates well with good outcome, and poor testing overestimates the incidence of fetal compromise. Given these results, we can fairly safely observe a growth-retarded fetus in utero with a high probability of fetal health at delivery. These studies do not predict developmental and neurologic state on long-term follow-up. Here the findings may be more subtle than those such as Apgar score and pH used to determine neonatal state at birth.

Harvey et al.[9] have reported follow-up results on growth-retarded fetuses observed in utero with serial sonograms and delivered at or after 37 weeks. Follow-up evaluation after several years revealed neurologic deficits only in those children in whom onset of growth retardation was before 26 weeks. They did, however, find below-average height and weight on follow-up when onset of growth retardation was before 34 weeks. In a review of California birth records, Williams et al.,[6] found that with birth weight between 750 and 1,500 gm and weight below the 50th percentile, perinatal mortality increased with advancing gestational age. Also, with weight below the 10th percentile, no decrease in perinatal mortality was noted with longer duration in utero. Hence, continued growth in utero appears to be an important factor in the assessment of fetal health.

Dr. Mariona: Our inability to accurately diagnose IUGR may result in unnecessary and untimely intervention in these patients. It seems that may be happening in the management of this patient.

Dr. Bronsteen: Though not seen here, oligohydramnios may be another prognostic factor of fetal health with IUGR, although it seems to be a poor screen for this disorder.[10,11] Philipson et al.[11] found no increased morbidity when oligohydramnios was present as diagnosed by subjective criteria. Manning et al.,[10] however, did find increased morbidity when no pockets of fluid larger than 1 cm were seen.

In a recent review of studies that followed the progress of growth-retarded babies, Allen[12] states that term SGA babies experienced no higher incidence of major handicaps, but were at increased risk for minor cerebral dysfunction. On the other hand, preterm SGA babies did have an increased incidence of major handicaps. These studies do not always account for other factors such as birth asphyxia, degree of growth retardation, and socioeconomic status, which can also affect the results. Inference from these data is that it is preferential to observe growth-retarded infants in utero as long as antenatal heart rate testing is good, serial sonograms document fetal growth, and oligohydramnios is not present.

Dr. Mariona: Inclusion of biophysical profiles in the antenatal monitoring system may significantly improve the management of IUGR.

Dr. Sokol: It seems that our three perinatologists think that amniocentesis is not warranted at this time in this patient, but would rather follow this pregnancy with monitoring for continued fetal well-being. I agree.

> The pregnancy was managed conservatively, with bed rest and fetal movement recording. Biweekly nonstress tests were all reactive. At 37 weeks gestation by the first ultrasound study, a third ultrasound examination was performed. Biparietal diameter and femur length were consistent with 34 weeks gestation (i.e., 3 weeks growth deceleration compared with the initial study). The abdominal circumference was consistent with 33 weeks. The head circumference/abdominal circumference ratio was 1.5 SD above the mean. The fluid volume remained normal, and the placental grade was I.
>
> Inasmuch as fetal growth was demonstrated, it was decided not to effect delivery until 38 weeks gestation. However, 2 days later there was premature rupture of the membranes, with clear fluid. Contractions began spontaneously, and a vigorous 2,268 gm female infant was delivered vaginally. No complications were experienced with labor or delivery. The fetal monitoring tracing was normal. Neonatal assessment was 36 to 38 weeks estimated gestational age and "mild growth retardation." The infant did well in the nursery.

Dr. Mariona: It should be noted that a 2,268 gm infant at 37 weeks is above the 10th percentile for weight and therefore does not meet the criterion for SGA (Denver criteria).

Dr. Dombrowski: For this patient, a 2,268 gm infant at 37 weeks may not be truly growth retarded, especially in respect to her stature and to the birth weights of her previous children, who were born at term. Women who are destined to deliver constitutionally small infants may have infants that are labeled SGA but who are really appropriately grown for their ethnic or genetic background. Conversely, there is currently no acceptable means to classify an infant as being growth retarded if the birth weight is more than 2,500 gm. Neonates who had a hostile uterine environment, even though born at the 50th percentile of weight, will not have attained their maximum intrauterine growth. Although these infants are not growth retarded by growth curves, they are actually small for their potential. An example is the dysmature post-term infant. These neonates may even be at more risk than those infants who are constitutionally small and classified as growth retarded but who experienced an optimal intrauterine environment.

DR. MARIONA: Other parameters that would be of interest in this case are umbilical blood gases at birth, the placental-fetal weight ratio, the fetal ponderal index, and the mother's weight gain after the initial visit at 20 weeks gestation.

Using a sea level growth chart, this infant's birth weight for gestational age was at the 15th percentile. The infant did well, and it is difficult to say whether she was in fact growth retarded. This history certainly points up the difficulties of appropriately defining IUGR.

PATIENT 2

A 33-year-old gravida 4 para 2 abortus 1 was referred for care at 28 weeks gestation by menstrual dates because of significant size for dates discrepancy. The patient had received prenatal care at a local clinic, with visits at 12, 16, 20, and 24 weeks. At 28 weeks gestation the uterine fundus was noted to be just at the level of the umbilicus, and the patient was referred to our institution for further evaluation. Review of her records revealed maternal weight gain of 14 lb, negative urine reactions for protein and glucose, and blood pressure between 90 and 110 mm Hg systolic and 60 and 70 mm Hg diastolic. Fundal heights were not recorded, and fetal heart tones were only listed as "present." The VDRL was nonreactive, hematocrit was 36%, rubella titer 1:16, and blood type 0+. Results of a urine pregnancy test at 6 weeks menstrual age were positive.

The patient's medical history was remarkable only for appendectomy at age 16 years. Obstetric history revealed a voluntary interruption of pregnancy as a teenager, followed by two term deliveries (birth weights 3,232 and 3,459 gm) 2 and 5 years ago. The patient smoked half a pack of cigarettes per day and consumed alcohol only occasionally. Pertinent findings at examination included weight 124 lb and height 5 ft 4 inches. Blood pressure at initial exam was 100/70 mm Hg. Pulmonary and cardiac values were normal. The uterus was soft and nontender, with a fundal height 21 cm. Fetal heart tones were 150 by fetoscope. The cervix was 25% effaced and fingertip dilated. No fluid was noted in the vagina.

DR. BRONSTEEN: Common in tertiary centers is the referral of a patient with poor menstrual dates or size for dates discrepancy. This patient presented a similar dilemma because of regular but suboptimal antenatal care. Important gestational landmarks such as fundal height measurements and auscultation of fetal heart tones with a fetoscope were not recorded at any of the visits. Thus based on results of her earlier examinations we cannot rule out incorrect dates. However, the positive reaction of a urine pregnancy test at 6 weeks, if not false positive, is suggestive of the validity of the dates and of significant growth retardation. Because of the size for dates difference, careful sonographic evaluation is indicated for dating and to rule out growth retardation or structural abnormalities.

Real time ultrasonography revealed a single fetus with biparietal diameter, femur length, and abdominal circumference consistent with 23 weeks gestation. The placenta was fundal and grade I, and there was decreased amniotic fluid, although the largest fluid pockets were more than 1 cm. No fetal anomalies were seen. The kidneys were not visualized because of fetal position; fetal bladder appeared normal.

The working diagnosis at this time was that this fetus probably was symmetrically growth retarded at 28 weeks gestation by menstrual dates and early positive pregnancy test results. However, it remained possible that this could simply be a case of incorrect menstrual dates, with an appropriately grown fetus.

DR. DOMBROWSKI: Symmetric growth retardation is relatively rare and is frequently associated with etiologic factors that as a whole are much more ominous than those causing asymmetric growth retardation.

DR. BRONSTEEN: The etiology of symmetric growth retardation in an otherwise healthy gravida points to the possibilities of a genetic abnormality or congenital infection. Various syndromes associated with IUGR include trisomies 13, 18, and 21, Turner's syndrome, and numerous other less common genetic abnormalities. Infectious agents are associated with IUGR in 10% of cases. The most common agents are the TORCH infections. However, this patient denied a history of febrile illnesses or contacts.

Because of the possibility of congenital abnormalities, amniocentesis was performed to obtain a fetal karyotype. A nonstress test performed at this time was not reactive; accelerations were only 5 to 10 beats per minute with fetal movements. The patient was placed on bed rest at home and instructed to keep a daily journal of fetal movements. Conservative management was planned for as long as fetal growth could be documented, as evaluated by serial ultrasound studies.

DR. SOKOL: I believe that management in this patient was not intensive enough. In the face of suspected IUGR and a nonreactive nonstress test, more intensive antepartum fetal assessment is warranted if indeed the gestational duration is 28 weeks. Given the positive early pregnancy test result, I think the actual management would be difficult to defend medicolegally. On the other hand, if the clinicians really believed that this was a previable fetus (23 weeks), then either the nonstress test should not have been done, because we would not intervene at 23 weeks, or the monitoring tracing obtained to "control" the amniocentesis should not have been interpreted like a nonstress test. There are no available formal criteria for nonstress test interpretation at 23 weeks.

> The karyotype was diagnostic of trisomy 13. Because of the uniformly severe prognosis of this disorder, an informed decision was made to terminate the pregnancy. Induction was accomplished by cervical ripening with laminaria, followed by prostaglandin suppositories. A 550 g male fetus was delivered with a gross appearance consistent with the diagnosis of trisomy 13. The neonate died several hours after delivery.

DR. BRONSTEEN: In our experience, antenatal diagnosis of growth retardation on the basis of genetic abnormalities is rarely made. Although amniocentesis is an invasive procedure, it can be essential for the diagnosis of genetic abnormalities, which is most helpful in avoiding cesarean delivery of an infant incapable of extrauterine life.

DR. MARIONA: In the presence of documented early second-trimester size for dates discrepancy, the invasiveness of amniocentesis is offset by the importance of information derived from its performance. At age 33 years the patient carries an inherent risk of approximately 1 in 600 for an infant with Down's syndrome and of approximately 1 in 300 for all genetic abnormalities. This compares favorably with the overall complication risk of approximately 1 in 200 for amniocentesis. We may speculate that if maternal screening of serum α-fetoprotein had been done the value may well have been below normal and therefore amniocentesis would have been performed at 16 weeks gestation, with resultant early diagnosis of trisomy 13.

CONCLUSION

It is clear that IUGR presents a problem to the clinician not only regarding management but also in diagnosis and etiology. Many growth-retarded fetuses are not diagnosed prior to birth. There is even difficulty in recognizing the growth-retarded neonate unless it also happens to be SGA.

Specific causes of growth retardation, such as infection, genetic abnormalities, hypertension, multiple gestations, structural abnormalities, maternal malnutrition, and toxins, can only be identified in a relatively small number of growth-retarded fetuses. Without knowledge of the cause it is impossible to develop or apply specific therapies. Our present level of sophistication in the treatment of growth retardation might be compared with that of the understanding and treatment of Rh disease in the early 1960s. We are only able to either give supportive therapy or effect early delivery when advantageous; definitive treatment is not yet feasible. It is likely that as our understanding of the mechanisms of growth retardation become more specific than simply diagnosing "uteroplacental insufficiency" in the majority of cases, then therapies for IUGR will become more definitive. Until that time, there will no doubt remain a wide dichotomy of opinions as to how to best manage this difficult and perplexing problem.

REFERENCES

1. Belizán JM, Villar J, Nardin JC, et al: Diagnosis of intrauterine growth retardation by a simple clinical method: Measurement of uterine height. *Am J Obstet Gynecol* 1978; 131:643.
2. Gross TL, Sokol RJ, Wilson MV, et al: Amniotic fluid phosphatidylglycerol: A potentially useful predictor of intrauterine growth retardation. *Am J Obstet Gynecol* 1981; 140:277.
3. Gross TL, Sokol RJ, Wilson MV, et al: Using ultrasound and amniotic fluid determinations to diagnose intrauterine growth retardation before birth: A clinical model. *Am J Obstet Gynecol* 1982; 143:265.
4. Perry CP, Harris RE, DeLemos RH, et al: Intrauterine growth retarded infants — Correlation of gestational age with maternal factors, mode of delivery, and perinatal survival. *Obstet Gynecol* 1976; 48:182.
5. Battaglia FC: Intrauterine growth retardation. *Am J Obstet Gynecol* 1970; 106:1103.
6. Williams RL, Creasy RK, Cunningham GC, et al: Fetal growth and perinatal viability in California. *Obstet Gynecol* 1982; 59:624.
7. Cetrulo CL, Freeman R: Bioelectric evaluation in intrauterine growth retardation. *Clin Obstet Gynecol* 1977; 20:979.
8. Lin CC, Devoe LD, River P, et al: Oxytocin challenge test and intrauterine growth retardation. *Am J Obstet Gynecol* 1981; 140:282.
9. Harvey D, Prince J, Bunton J, et al: Abilities of children who were small-for-gestational-age babies. *Pediatrics* 1982; 69:296.
10. Manning FA, Hill LM, Platt LD: Qualitative amniotic fluid volume determination by ultrasound: Antepartum detection of intrauterine growth retardation. *Am J Obstet Gynecol* 1981; 139:254.
11. Philipson EH, Sokol RJ, Williams T: Oligohydramnios: Clinical associations and predictive value for intrauterine growth retardation. *Am J Obstet Gynecol* 1983; 146:271.
12. Allen MC: Developmental outcome and followup of the small for gestational age infant. *Semin Perinatol* 1984; 8:123.

PART VI

Medicolegal

17

Malpractice Implications of Intrauterine Growth Retardation

Robert J. Sokol, M.D.
Mark I. Evans, M.D.

No discussion of any controversial medical topic is complete without addressing the issue of the attorney who knows why the physician "screwed up." Management of complicated obstetric problems fills the literature and has been source material for many textbooks, yet malpractice attorneys often have successfully reduced the practice of medicine to three words: standard of care. It is not surprising that most obstetricians believe, particularly with regard to complicated pregnancy management decisions, that there is simply no such thing. Nevertheless, certain guidelines do appear appropriate for the management of the potentially compromised pregnancy to reduce the risk of significant perinatal morbidity and mortality. However, and particularly with intrauterine growth retardation (IUGR), morbidity and mortality can never be completely eliminated. There will always be significant risk to the physician who manages "high-risk" pregnancies. There is always the custom of striving for best practice while avoiding the pitfall of malpractice. Clearly some actions taken by physicians are grossly incompetent and place mother and baby in substantial danger. We make no attempt to defend the indefensible. What we seek to attempt, however, is to generate guidelines that may reduce the likelihood of litigation. It must be understood that a guideline and a standard are not synonymous. A guideline is a pattern of action that can be deviated from in appropriate circumstances, whereas with a standard the physician risks censure by deviation.

With specific regard to IUGR, the compromised fetus dictates a higher level of awareness in physician management. Such a philosophy can reasonably be considered a standard. The implementation of such high awareness can be managed by following a set of guidelines. For example, it would seem that for the greatest liability protection, without having to apply it to every moderately suspect case, a policy of managing IUGR similar to that adopted by some obstetricians for vaginal breech delivery in multiple gestations is appropriate:

1. Observe closely.
2. Allow the pregnancy to progress so long as — and only so long as — all parameters are completely normal.
3. Intervene at the first hint of a problem.

Such a philosophy would appear to be both medically prudent and also most legally defensible. We would, however, expect a high rate of cesarean section, with concomitant shifting of risk from fetus to mother. Although it is inevitable that some deleterious maternal outcomes will be generated, a relatively healthy mother is less likely to sustain permanent injury than is a compromised fetus. There is high probability of litigation with any poor maternal outcome, but the relative paucity of such bad maternal outcomes argues for maternal risk rather than adverse infant outcome, with greater probability of a suit.

FOUNDATION OF MALPRACTICE

Much of the medicolegal terminology used today can be traced to *Boyce v Brown* (Arizona 1938),[1] in which the legal elements of malpractice were established:

1. The physician fails to possess the requisite skill in learning or fails to apply it.
2. The physician does something the standard forbids or fails to do something the standard requires.
3. The standard must be shown by affirmative evidence (i.e., testimony of experts).
4. Negligence is never assumed by the mere fact of an unsuccessful result but affirmatively proved by testimony.
5. Negligence must be established by expert testimony unless it is so grossly apparent that a lay person would recognize it.
6. Expert testimony by another physician that he or she would have done otherwise is not sufficient to establish malpractice unless the course of therapy followed deviated from the approved standard.

The medicolegal implications of high-risk medical practice raise several areas of concern. As has been well summarized by Nocon and Coolman,[2] most legitimate lawsuits are based on failure to follow the standard of care, obtain proper informed consent, diagnose, treat properly, or maintain adequate records.

Standard of Care

A critical issue with regard to malpractice and IUGR is that the standard of care, even in the most ethereal setting, is hotly debated. A good attorney can easily find a well-respected physician to argue virtually any reasonable point of view. However, court decisions as far back as 50 years argued that the term "standard of care" defines a duty to use "reasonable" care as would be expected of a "prudent" person. Failure to offer such care, which is a substantial factor in causing harm, can be considered negligence.[1]

In this framework the profession of expert witness was created. One major problem in today's malpractice crisis is that some physicians, including some with impeccable credentials, have made plaintiff's testimony a major source of income. Medical organizations, such as the American College of Obstetricians and Gynecologists, have begun to debate criteria for "expert" witnesses to identify to juries those witnesses noted to be "professional witnesses."

Informed Consent

In the past it was common for patients to be subjected to a variety of potential treatments, often without the faintest clue as to why.[3] This is still the case in many countries, although total failure of informed consent is a diminishing problem in the United States. To a degree, malpractice fear has had a positive effect on medical care, if only in that no longer are patients led blindly down a therapeutic path without at least having been offered an explanation of the options. In discussions with ethical and legal experts from other societies, however, such principles have not been adopted universally. In the United States the overabundance of paperwork necessary to perform any procedure has eliminated this issue in the vast majority of cases.

Failure to Diagnose

Diagnostic abilities among physicians have and will always vary. Nevertheless, one important distinction obvious to physicians but ignored by lawyers is that tertiary center capabilities should not be expected of all primary care physicians. Nevertheless, it is often tertiary center physicians who point accusing fingers at community physicians who have not been able to make some esoteric diagnosis.

Such a double standard is truly unfair, as has been evidenced in a large number of lawsuits. The greatest liability, however, is most often reserved for those cases in which a diagnosis clearly should have been possible by primary physicians without assistance of a highly trained subspecialist. Anecdotally, it often seems that academic physicians are more likely to be sued because they see a higher proportion of high-risk and indigent patients.

Failure to Treat

The same type of philosophic approach exists for treatment as for diagnosis. For IUGR the major treatment concerns are surveillance, timing, and method of delivery. Thus, although potential novel intrauterine therapies are possible (as discussed in previous chapters), the option of performing a cesarean section in a patient who appears to be at risk should clearly be available. A phenomenal number of lawsuits have been based strictly on whether cesarean delivery was offered to the patient at the appropriate time. Particularly in high-risk situations there will always be debate as to when is the "appropriate time" for an intervention.

Failure to Maintain Adequate Records

Perhaps the single most preventable cause of litigation is failure to document records adequately. Probably the most important advice for obstetricians in high-risk situations is never chart a problem that you don't address.

Conclusions

The specific application of these principles to the management of IUGR confirms the obvious: a good outcome is the best defense against a potential lawsuit. However, with the compromised fetus a good outcome is not always possible despite the best efforts of highly trained personnel. The defense of a poor outcome rests primarily on the following:

1. A thorough understanding of what the options were.
2. The compulsiveness of the physician managing the case.
3. The direct evidence of patient input.
4. Documentation of what was done.

In a known compromised fetus, prolonged pregnancy engenders particularly high risk for a malpractice suit. With any evidence of IUGR, perinatal risks in prolonged pregnancy appear to be substantially higher, and the chance for something to go wrong is vastly increased.[4–7] Given the body of literature on this subject, a bad outcome under such circumstances could realistically be construed as failure to observe the patient's best interests.

CASE REPORT

> A 16-year-old gravida 1 para 0 black woman first came for prenatal care at approximately 24 weeks by dates. Her past medical and gynecologic history was normal, and family history was noncontributory. Her height was 5 ft 3 inches, and weight 106 lb at the first visit. General physical examination including vital signs yielded completely normal findings. Fundal height was 24 cm. Repeat visits were made every 3 weeks. Fundal height was 26 cm at 27 weeks, 28 cm at 30 weeks, 30 cm at 32 weeks, 31 cm at 35 weeks, 32 cm at 38 weeks, 32 cm at 40 weeks, and 32 cm at 41 weeks.
>
> The patient had an unripe cervix at term, and spontaneous labor began at 41.5 weeks. Fundal height was 31 cm. On admission the cervix was 2 cm dilated and 60% effaced, and station was −3. Membranes were ruptured artificially, revealing a small amount of amniotic fluid stained with thick meconium. Labor continued to progress at approximately 1 cm per hour. After one and one-half hours of second-stage labor a 2,500 gm female infant was delivered, with Apgar score 2 at 1 minute and 5 at 5 minutes. A DeLee trap was used for intrapartum suction. Pediatricians were present at the delivery. Meconium was aspirated from the lungs. No cord pH was obtained. In the nursery the baby did reasonably well, with no evidence of seizure activity. At 4 years of age the child's development was believed to be lagging. A lawsuit was filed.

Evaluation of the "facts" of this case reveals many areas of poor care that would pave the way for successful litigation without even the need to prove cause and effect. Certain teenagers are at higher than average risk for a fetus with IUGR, which may have been detectable in this case before term. The lack of fetal growth over a 6-week period cannot be considered normal, and by any standard deserved obstetric concern and evaluation. Nevertheless, no common prenatal testing such as ultrasonography and electronic fetal monitoring was used. Without any evidence of such investigative studies, a fetus could quite logically be expected to be at considerable risk without detection. Because of the lack of objective data, the obstetrician is put on the defensive a priori. In the postdates period, particularly, fetuses with IUGR are known to be at significantly higher risk for fetal damage that could have occurred before the onset of labor and would not be expected to be manifested in labor. Even though an external labor tracing pattern may be within normal limits, the infant is not necessarily normal.

The documentation of meconium, particularly with oligohydramnios, is considered ominous by many authorities. In our opinion, regardless of the time in gestation, the finding of meconium-stained amniotic fluid clearly warrants intensive observation, with internal electronic monitoring and early delivery. The lack of use of available technology in a high-risk situation, both antepartum and intrapartum, bodes poorly for the defense of a bad outcome. Regardless of the arguments against both routine ultrasonography and electronic fetal monitoring,[8,9] obstetricians who do not rely on available technology can expect a bad outcome in a malpractice suit. While not necessarily an appropriate medical judgment, the conclusion is a legal fact of life. Finally, failure to obtain a fetal cord blood sample is a serious logistic error on the part of the obstetrician, because normal pH is often the best evidence against perinatal asphyxia.

It could be anticipated, given the series of flaws in this case, that a judgment for millions of dollars would be awarded the plaintiff. Few obstetricians have difficulty with the concept of awarding patients for gross negligence. The situation becomes more frustrating when cases with only minor elements of questionable deviation from optimal care are seen and such judgments are awarded anyway.

SUMMARY

Given the clearly understood high morbidity and fetal mortality in the postdates period and in the IUGR pregnancy, it is our recommendation that pregnancies with IUGR are at such risk that they should virtually never be allowed to continue into the postdates period. We recognize that this is not a universally held opinion. When the mother has a ripe cervix, the mature growth-retarded fetus should be delivered regardless of actual gestational age. When the cervix is ripe and the immature fetus with IUGR is stable, close observation is warranted. With an unripe maternal cervix the mature fetus with IUGR can also be observed closely, but the pregnancy should not be allowed to go beyond 40 weeks. We hold these opinions even though much of the current literature argues for a more expectant management of the postdates pregnancy. There is room for debate about the merits of induction versus surveillance when the fetus is appropriate for gestational age, and even the two authors of this chapter disagree about such management. However, the IUGR pregnancy does not fit the category of those that can be watched. It is clear that surveillance techniques are not as reliable in the postdates period, and we believe this is particularly true of the IUGR pregnancy.[10]

A major problem arises when the maternal cervix is unripe. Management is controversial not only because of the malpractice crisis. It is our belief that the IUGR pregnancy should not continue past term because, among other medical issues, the high morbidity and mortality rate in these cases is virtually impossible to differentiate from that in cases of "theoretical mismanagement."

Although the management of the preterm or term IUGR pregnancy is still logically open to debate, the preponderance of evidence suggesting poor outcomes in postdates IUGR would tend to have established a standard against which poor outcomes will be unfavorably reviewed. Such a trend in the legal precedent will make it virtually impossible to test new treatment methods that might allow pregnancies to continue under those circumstances. The same trend has been seen in several other areas, including midforceps extraction.[11] There is no proper scientific response under these circumstances, and it remains likely that legal precedence will become as much a part of obstetric decision making in complicated pregnancies as any advances in science are.

REFERENCES

1. *Boyce v Brown,* 51 Ariz 416, 77 P2d 455 (1938).
2. Nocon JJ, Coolman DA: Perinatal malpractice: Risks and prevention. *J Reprod Med* 1987; 32(2):83.
3. Fletcher JC, Beng K, Tranoy KE; Ethical aspects of medical genetics, in Beng K (ed): *Medical Genetics: Past, Present, Future*. New York, Alan R Liss, 1985, pp 511–524.
4. Lin CC, Evans MI: Introduction, in Lin CC, Evans MI (eds): *Intrauterine Growth Retardation: Pathophysiology and Clinical Management*. New York, McGraw-Hill Publishing Co, 1984, pp 1–15.
5. Cario GM: Conservative management of prolonged pregnancy using fetal heart rate monitoring only: A prospective study. *Br J Obstet Gynaecol* 1984; 91:23.
6. Leveno KJ, Quirk JG Jr, Cunningham FG, et al: Prolonged pregnancy. I: Observations covering the cases of fetal distress. *Am J Obstet Gynecol* 1984; 150:465.
7. Yeh SY, Read JA: Management of post-term pregnancy in a large obstetric population. *Obstet Gynecol* 1986; 60:282.
8. *Diagnostic Ultrasound Imaging in Pregnancy*. Rockville, Md, US Department of Health and Human Services, NIH Publication 84–667, 1984.
9. Banta HD, Thacker SB: Policies toward medical technology: The case of elective fetal monitoring. *Am J Public Health* 1979; 69:941.
10. Devoe LD, Sholl JS: Postdates pregnancy: Assessment of fetal risk and obstetric management. *J Reprod Med* 1983; 28:576.
11. Richardson DA, Evans MI, Cibils LA: Midforceps: A critical review. *Am J Obstet Gynecol* 1983; 145:621.

Index

G

H

I